SEX,
MA
AND THE CHURCH

"Muriel Porter has written a lively, scholarly, and courageous book on the history of the Church's changing attitudes to sexuality. She challenges the notion that the Church has preserved a uniform, pristine, and unchanging position on matters of sexual ethics and sexual expression, showing how the Church has been compelled more than once to change its mind.

"The conclusion is a powerful and provocative one: if the Church can change its position in the past, it may well need to do so again, given the different context of sexuality, particularly in the light of contraception and the modern phenomenon of homosexuality. Basic Christian ethics – love, care, commitment – can be expressed in more ways than the traditional model of marriage and the nuclear family. The Church is encouraged to think again and rearticulate Christian ethics in new ways more relevant to modern society.

"This is a very important book. Beneath the challenge to the Church to reconsider so-called 'traditional' values lies a deeper challenge to the dualism that has pervaded so much of Western Christianity. Dr Porter shows that the denial of the body – bodily pleasure and bodily intimacy – is a serious flaw in the Western tradition, and that the recovery of a truly integrated and holistic anthropology is vital for the survival of the Church as it enters the twenty-first century.

"This book is eminently readable, grounded in sound scholarly research, and written with lively vigor and imagination. It is a must for those seeking a Christianity that is no longer dualistic or anti-life: a Christianity genuinely grounded in the incarnation."

DOROTHY A. LEE
Professor of New Testament
United Faculty of Theology, Melbourne

For Patrick and Emily,
in the hope that their generation
might experience a more generous and loving Church

SEX, MARRIAGE, AND THE CHURCH

Patterns of Change

MURIEL PORTER

Dove

An imprint of HarperCollins*Publishers*

A Dove publication
An imprint of HarperCollins*Religious*
(ACN 005 677 805)
A member of the HarperCollins*Publishers* (Australia) Pty Ltd group
22–24 Joseph Street
North Blackburn, Victoria 3130, Australia

First published 1996
Designed by William Hung
Cover design by William Hung
Cover painting: "Angel Spying on Adam and Eve," (1947–1948), by Arthur Boyd
Typeset in Perpetua by J&M Typesetting
Printed in Australia by Griffin Paperbacks

National Library of Australia Cataloguing-in-Publication data:
Porter, Muriel, 1948– .
   Sex, marriage, and the church: patterns of change.

   Bibliography.
   Includes index.
   ISBN 1 86371 597 5.

   1. Interpersonal relations – Religious aspects –
   Christianity. 2. Intimacy – Religious aspects –
   Christianity. 3. Sex – Religious aspects – Christianity.
   4. Marriage – Religious aspects – Christianity. I. Title.

261.8357

Our thanks go to those who have given us permission to reproduce copyright
material in this book. All rights of copyright holders are reserved. Particular
sources of print material are acknowledged in the text. Every effort has been
made to contact the copyright holders of print material, and the publisher
welcomes communication from any copyright holder from whom permission was
inadvertently not gained.

CONTENTS

FOREWORD ■

One of the most important books of our era is undoubtedly *The Structure of Scientific Revolutions* by Thomas Kuhn, the science historian. For Kuhn, a paradigm is "an entire constellation of beliefs, values, techniques which are shared by the members of a particular community," and the power of a paradigm lies in the largely unconscious way we inhabit it or take it for granted. We tend to treat the world view that we have inherited as having absolute and eternal validity, and we are profoundly shaken when it is challenged. Revolutions in thinking and behaving are extremely painful experiences to undergo and they are invariably characterized by bitterness, hostility and a pervasive sense of disorientation.

Though Kuhn applied his theory mainly to the world of science, he has provided historians of culture with an invaluable tool for assessing human social and moral evolution, and here the pains of transition and change are even harder fought than in the field of science. Most of us assume that the values and attitudes we have inherited are self-evident and unchanging and, like Molière's M. Jourdain, who was surprised to discover that he'd been speaking prose for more than forty years without knowing it, we find it difficult to accept what might appear to be the arbitrary nature of our own beliefs.

Hans Küng, in his sweeping narrative study *Christianity*, uses Kuhn's typology to study the history of the Christian Faith. He says that, so far, it has expressed itself in five paradigms in its 2000-year history and a sixth paradigm is beginning to emerge in our own day. Those who are profoundly rooted in one of the expressions of Christianity find it difficult to believe that there is much validity in any of the others, but a study of the evidence soon demonstrates the provisionality of all systems and shows that they are inescapably related to their context and the influence of individuals of genius. The Christian Church has endured many revolutions with consequent pain and distress as well as renewed creativity and commitment.

Muriel Porter's important book is a scholarly study of a paradigm shift in the Christian understanding of sexuality. The medieval Christian world view saw sexuality as a moral disease for which the only real cure was celibacy. Celibacy was the eschatological ideal that had Christianity enthralled for centuries, however dishonored it was in practice. If virginity was the cure for the disease of sex, then marriage offered a licensed palliative "for those that had not the gift of continence." However, this concession to be allowed to marry rather than to burn with lust was not offered to the clergy. For them the eschatological ideal was compulsory. Thus was set the scene for one of the great set-piece struggles of the Reformation, carefully documented in this important study.

Muriel Porter's intention in writing this book is not simply to revisit an old battle but to find ammunition for a new one. Paradigm shifts are painful, and the shift to a married clergy and a new and more positive evaluation of marriage itself was not easily won. Dr Porter believes, I think correctly, that the Christian Church is on the cusp of another revolution in its thinking about, and attitudes toward, sexuality. The debate about the moral status of sexual activity outside marriage is already fierce in the Church and it is not likely to subside. By offering us invaluable insights into a previous revolution this book will give us the courage to negotiate our own.

The Most Revd Richard Holloway,
Bishop of Edinburgh,
Primus of the Scottish Episcopal Church

PREFACE

The sixteenth-century Reformation debate over the marriage of the clergy marked a crucial sea change in the Christian understanding of human sexuality. It was the point at which the Church finally began to abandon its long obsession with asceticism, and moved toward a radically new acceptance of the goodness of sex and human intimacy, and even a reappraisal of the worth of women.

That journey is by no means complete, four hundred years later. It has been a painfully slow journey, and many people have suffered from the Church's narrow and restrictive views along the way. Still today they suffer: in all the churches – single people, young people, and homosexuals who cannot fit into simplistic categories and rules; in the Catholic Church specifically – couples who wish to practice contraception or to remarry in Church, and priests who long for the companionship and fulfillment of marriage.

That the Anglican, Protestant and Orthodox churches all now accept divorce, remarriage and contraception is linked with the continuing development in those churches of the theology of sex and marriage, made possible by their acceptance of a married clergy. The very experience of marriage and intimacy on the part of their theological leaders has facilitated these further developments. That such developments have been nevertheless slow-moving is possibly connected to the fact that, until very recently, clergy and theologians have been almost exclusively male. It will be interesting for future historians to see whether the rise of feminine influence in church leadership has any major impact on the pace of change in these areas of intimacy, which are of such importance to women's lives.

My doctoral study of the little-known Reformation clerical marriage debate made it abundantly clear to me that the Christian Church made a radical about-face on human sexuality at that time. The abandonment of the ideal of asceticism in favour of an ideal of marriage was profound and quite fundamental, and opened the way to a seldom-recognised continuing process of change. The sum total of that change stands as a continual indictment of those who would claim that the Christian Church has always had — and therefore always must have — one set of rules for sexual conduct.

The purpose of this book is unashamedly polemical. Faced with the needs of modern society and, indeed, of modern churchgoers, theologians and Scripture scholars have been grappling with the problem of developing new doctrinal standards in this area. Again and again they are confronted by conservative forces insisting that there is no freedom to change, because the Church's tradition mitigates against it. This book presents incontrovertible evidence that the Church has changed its mind, and changed it often. There are no tablets of stone. There is freedom to change.

Given the limitations of length and the purposes for which it was written, this book does not purport to provide comprehensive coverage in every possible area of such a major issue. It focuses in most detail on the clerical marriage debate of the sixteenth century, because that debate ushered in the most fundamental of all changes in the Christian understanding of sexuality. This book is not the definitive summary of all the facets of the Church's history in the areas of sex and marriage, however; it has had to be selective. Nor is it primarily a study of either theology or Scripture, but of history. But I believe it offers a fair and balanced coverage of the key areas of debate. It seeks to be scholarly, but also accessible to the thoughtful cleric or layperson seeking a solid historical background for important contemporary debates on human sexuality.

For obvious reasons, the book is mainly concerned with the changing Christian rules governing heterosexual activity, principally related to marriage. It is only very recently that the mainstream churches have been publicly confronted with the need to reconsider issues relating to homosexuality. But I hope it will become apparent that the historical evidence presented here offers a constructive way forward for the churches' approach to homosexuality as well.

For the post-Reformation period, this book uses the experience of the Anglican Church as its main source. This is not simply because I am an Anglican, and feel more at home within my own Communion! The Anglican Church, with its traditional "via media" approach, provides an excellent case study at most points. Because of accidents of history, the Reformation debate about clergy marriage was most protracted in the Church of England (Mother Church of Anglicanism), and therefore provides evidence of the nature of that debate in more significant detail than would be found in other reformed churches. It follows from its continuing reliance on its Catholic heritage that the Anglican Church has leaned strongly toward Rome in its teaching on divorce in particular. Moreover it has, in recent decades, finally broken that particular nexus, and moved to a position close to that of the Protestant churches, with whom it shares much other common ground. This experience, however, might well have something to offer the Church of Rome, should it choose to re-examine its own position. The Anglican Church is also the Church that pioneered Christian acceptance of artificial contraception, and may yet have something to offer Rome on that score as well. Further, the Anglican Church has a strong international identity through the worldwide Anglican Communion, and so offers insights that are applicable around the Western world.

———————————■———————————

I thank the many people who have urged me to publish the results of my research in this area, and who have supported me in this project. In particular, I thank those who have also been kind enough to read the drafts of this book, and who have offered constructive criticism – specially my husband Brian, and my friends the Revd Dr Graeme Garrett, the Revd Professor Dorothy Lee and the Revd Canon Graeme Rutherford. I am grateful to my employer, the Royal Melbourne Institute of Technology, for providing generous study leave for the writing of the book. As the wife of a priest, my heartfelt thanks must be offered up too for those brave sixteenth-century reformers and their wives, who endured much personal abuse for their championing of the good of marriage. The Church owes them an incalculable debt.

1

CERTAINTY
AT ANY PRICE?

In the last decades of the twentieth century, the pace of change in modern Western societies is nowhere more evident than in questions of sexual morality. Advances in medical technology since the 1960s have ensured that, for the first time in human history, fertility can be controlled easily and with relative safety. The age-old fear of out-of-wedlock pregnancy has been effectively wiped from the human psyche, creating a revolution in our perception of the possible consequences of extramarital relationships. While the threat of HIV/AIDS has in more recent years tempered the earlier "live-and-let-live" attitude of the 1970s, the fact remains that the most powerful brake on unrestrained sexual activity since human life began has largely been lifted.

The Christian churches, by and large, have failed to come to grips with the full implications of this far-reaching social change. They have allowed themselves to be trapped into continuing to espouse a "pre-Pill" moral code that has little relevance anymore for society in general. Theologians and biblical scholars have agonized over the issues but, perhaps through a failure of nerve, too often they have ended up supporting the old order. For in this issue above all others, the conservatives in all the churches manage to maintain a powerful stranglehold. They do so generally in the name of offering "certainty," but one unstated agenda can often be detected – the desire to uphold Christians, or certain groups of Christians, as a "holier than thou" caste in

1

modern society. "The scandal of the Cross these days is that a young Christian male cannot sleep with his girlfriend," as one clergyman has put it. The upholding of a separate caste or castes via sexual rules and standards is in fact an ancient practice in the Christian Church.

Recently, the Anglican Diocese of Melbourne, like many others around the world, debated sexual morality in its synod. The debate was framed as an issue of "certainty." The synod was asked to agree that the uncertainty in modern society over standards of sexual morality had "destructive consequences for individuals, families and the community at large." In the name of offering "certainty," the synod was asked to re-affirm "the Christian standard of faithfulness within marriage and chastity outside marriage." It called on all Christians, and particularly Christian leaders, by their example, to "teach and encourage the traditional understanding of sexual morality."[1]

The implicit background to that debate, and doubtless to the many like it that have occupied the councils of the churches these past decades, is the assumption that there is one, and one only, Christian understanding of sexuality. Briefly, the Christian norm being espoused is the exclusive lifelong sexual union between a heterosexual couple formally married. Outside that norm, there is no room for sexual activity. In other words, it is acceptable either to be married or celibate (meaning not just unmarried, but chaste), and nothing else. And legal marriage is portrayed as the ideal lifestyle for Christian people. Outside it, the dangers and difficulties of leading an undefiled life are supreme. This is the way it has always been, and the way things should remain, it is argued – as if these particular rules and standards of sexual morality had been engraved by God on tablets of stone at the beginning of the world.[2]

But the simple historical truth is that they were not. There are few if any such absolutes in Christian moral teaching that have endured over the centuries. The Church has changed its mind often on issues of sexuality. Some of those changes were minor; some were major, to the extent of being nothing less than paradigm shifts. In particular, the debate over the marriage of the clergy during the sixteenth-century Reformation charts in considerable detail the nuances of one major paradigm shift in Christian understandings of sexuality. The changes brought about by that far-reaching development – a married clergy in the reformed churches – have in fact created the basis of the sexual morality and doctrine now upheld substantially by all the churches, including the Roman Catholic. It is the changed pattern that is now the norm; we have forgotten that there was ever any other. To compound our misunderstanding, we tend to read back into Scripture and other texts the presuppositions we bring from our post-Reformation perspective. We need humbly to bear in mind novelist L. P. Hartley's pithy comment: "The past is a foreign country; they do things differently there."[3]

The sixteenth-century debate about married clergy had enormous ramifications. The most striking result was that, in significant parts of the Christian Church, for the first time since the earliest Christian decades a married clergy was accepted as standard, rather than, at best, a barely tolerated aberration or, at worst, a scandal to the faithful. A moment's reflection on this about-face will suggest how great a change in the Church's attitude to sexuality, marriage and the role of women must have been involved. However, this debate and its implications have been almost entirely ignored by scholars, despite the intense interest shown by historians and theologians in all aspects of the Reformation over the past 400 years. Its theological and ecclesiological importance has been scarcely recognised at all.[4]

Perhaps this neglect has obtained because a married clergy became so much a part of the fabric of life in Protestant churches that it was taken for granted, and its significance was quickly forgotten. Curiously, even Catholic historians and theologians who, in recent years, have argued for a married clergy, have ignored the experience of Protestantism almost entirely. The end result has been that a key debate that acted as a bridge between medieval and contemporary views on sex and marriage in all the churches has been overlooked. With it, the opportunity of understanding how the Church is able to change its mind in such a major and fundamental area has been lost.

This is the key issue of this book. The Reformation debate about clerical marriage is endlessly fascinating in itself, but its major importance for contemporary scholarship lies in its ability to assist the contemporary Church's coming to grips with a current paradigm shift of similar proportions. That is the major reason why the sixteenth-century debate about clerical marriage is the central issue here, quite apart from the fact that the story of that critical struggle deserves to be far more widely known. It is pivotal to any historical discussion about attitudes to sex and marriage.

As we will discover in the succeeding chapters, clerical marriage was a contentious issue in England from the 1520s, during the reign of Henry VIII, until the 1580s, the latter part of the reign of Elizabeth I. It was not finally legalized in England until 1604, decades after it had become fully accepted in the reformed Continental churches.[5] The changing fortunes of the Reformation in England over that long period of time were partly the reason for the reformed Church of England's slowness to adopt a married clergy wholeheartedly, as we shall see. But because it was so protracted a struggle in England, historians are fortunate to have at their disposal the weapons in the propaganda war, in the form of the many polemical tracts published by the promoters of clerical marriage. These documents, read carefully, allow us to trace the theological and ecclesiological reasons why the reformers insisted so powerfully on promoting a married priesthood.

For they did not present these arguments lightly, or offer a married priesthood as a convenient "optional extra" of the Reformation. They paid a high price for their insistence on this particular reform, for there was no other single aspect of their reforming efforts which stimulated anything like the personal opprobrium that fell on them when they defended clerical matrimony. To their opponents, the reformers were simply lecherous men who wanted to indulge, even flaunt, their lusts publicly. To devout Catholics at the time, a married priest was a contradiction in terms, a man who had committed a sexual sin worse than adultery and close to incest. From the standpoint of Protestantism, as verified by historical research, the first generation of married priests, both on the Continent and in England, were mostly godly, clean-living and honest men, who did not deserve the outrageous slurs on their character they received. The bitterness of the vitriol on both sides, however, alerts us to the significance of this issue, which after all plumbs the depths of complex attitudes to human sexuality. The debate about priestly marriage, then, was not just an academic debate over a point of theology but rather, like the debate about women's ordination in our own time, a deeply personal and complex issue involving a reexamination of such fundamental concepts as the nature of priesthood, sacred power, holiness and anthropology.

A study of this particular debate, and the way in which it changed the Western view of sex and marriage, has much to teach the modern world. When I first began to study this area, I assumed that the reformers' commitment to a married clergy came directly from a new and higher view of sex and marriage, and even of the role of women. I was initially puzzled to discover no such thing. In many ways their views in these areas were not very different to those of their contemporaries on the other side of the debate. In itself, that is not actually so very surprising, for they were, after all, men of their own time. But this acknowledgment forced me to look for the real reasons that drove their passionate commitment.

I discovered that what lay behind the struggle was an over-riding concern to transform the Church and, through it, society. A married priesthood was not only a means to an end – even though most of the reformers at heart believed that it was a flawed means to an end – but an important symbol for this wider struggle. The changed view about human nature, and specifically about women, sex and marriage that this debate helped in no small measure to inaugurate, was an unexpected, though happy, outcome.

But to reach that unintended result – and, on the way, the intended outcome of offering a troubled society a more realistic pattern of life – the reformers had to compromise. They did not say this explicitly, but it is implicit in their arguments. To a man they upheld the ideal not of a married priesthood but of a celibate, and specifically chaste, one. To them the danger of defilement still hovered over all sexual activity, even in marriage. But to a man they recognized the need for what was, to them, a compromise attitude to priesthood, sex and marriage in order to achieve their overall aims. Their courage in embarking on such a compromise for the overall good meant that a new and better theological understanding of fundamental human issues became possible. In a sense, we could say that they did the right thing for the wrong reasons, or at least for reasons we might reject. But the end result vindicated that courageous decision.

What has that got to say to Christians in the last years of the twentieth century? Perhaps we need to travel down a different road, even while we debate the landscape, rather than remaining at the crossroads arguing. The Church at present seems to be debating at the junction, while society in general heads off, leaderless, down a road we, in the Church, are too nervous to take.

It is not that we are not fully aware of the direction of that road. Our leaders might take refuge in proclaiming old patterns of morality, claiming them immutable; but ordinary church members are fully aware of the extent of change in contemporary family patterns. They count among their friends and family divorced people, remarried people, sole parents, de facto couples, openly gay people. Some church members are divorced, remarried, sole parents, gay, though research suggests that such people, feeling the Church's general hostility, quickly move out of church membership.[6]

At the fringes there is, however, direct involvement with the churches. Clergy today conduct weddings for very few virgins. In fact, they are no longer surprised if couples already share a common address when they come for interview. Whether this is right or wrong, it is a simple statement of fact, and the Church must learn how to deal with it constructively rather than merely long for the return of a golden age when the only people who indulged in sexual activity were married heterosexual couples. The problem is of course that the golden age is a myth. Premarital sex was not invented in the "swinging '60s"; it just came out of the closet, where it had been for nearly a century. Where once young people made love under bushes or in the back seat of the family car, and hoped and prayed no pregnancy would result, today's young people set up house together, and have little to fear from unwanted pregnancy.

They also have little to fear from community disapproval! An Australian Bureau of Statistics survey of 1992 found that 56 percent of couples admitted to living together before marriage, compared with 16 percent in 1975. A majority of the population thought such "trial marriages" to be a good idea, including significant numbers of people who were regular churchgoers.[7] Presumably these figures refer precisely to couples who actually set up home together in some recognizable form, and do not count the other couples who, while not actually living together, nevertheless experience full sexual activity within their premarital relationship. The Australian pattern would be repeated all over modern Western society, in which premarital sex is readily and publicly accepted as a reality of life. This level of acceptance is a profound change that should not be underestimated, and a change that is clearly linked to – even caused by – the invention of safe and reliable forms of contraception. The implications for the churches' teaching are enormous, and must not be swept under the carpet with a superficial call for "certainty."[8] Similarly, there is a growing liberalism in attitudes in society to homosexuality and divorce,[9] which cannot be ignored.

The calls for a return to a simple but rigid standard of either marriage or celibacy in fact reflect a call not to an ancient Christian standard but to a relatively modern standard imposed by a wide range of factors, of which Christian teaching was only one. Historians of marriage practice point out that patterns of sexual restraint regarded as normative by our society are in fact relatively recent in origin. John R. Gillis, author of a definitive study of British marriage since medieval times, has argued that the period 1890 to 1960 – the period our generation regards as normative – actually imposed the most severe restraints on sexual activity within the past 400 years.[10]

In our culture this was the period of one of the highest levels of marriage of all time. By the middle of this century, only about 5 percent of women did not marry at some time during their life, in marked contrast to the 15 percent of those women born in the second half of last century who remained single. The emergence this century of the overwhelming expectation that everyone be married was responsible for creating the "spinster" and, to a lesser degree, the "bachelor," who were regarded as failures and even despised as "unnatural." As a consequence, only a few years ago a powerful dividing line existed in our society between the world of the married and the world of the single. The relatively recent invention of the so-called "traditional wedding," with its most powerful symbol of the white dress and veil, marked that divide. Brides in earlier centuries – and the first decades of this century – generally wore street clothes (though usually their best street clothes). Only brides from the upper classes could afford special wedding finery, in any case. From the 1930s, however, the white bridal gown became almost universal, emphasizing the "feminine purity and virtuous womanhood" of the virgin bride.[11] Those of us now middle-aged or older grew up in this pattern of expectation, knowing no other; it has deeply colored our thinking.

But the marriage practice of the first half of this century is, historically, something of an aberration. The current fluid situation, where there is no longer a clear distinction between the world of the married and that of the single, is far closer to older patterns of lifestyle.

Historians generally date modern marriage practices only from the middle of the seventeenth century. This was the time when, particularly in the growing middle classes, the notion of the marital relationship as the place of fulfillment of emotional and spiritual needs began to develop. The growth of this conjugal ideal was influenced strongly by radical puritanism – of which more later – and was for a long time a controversial notion, not widely accepted until the nineteenth century. But the seventeenth century was also a time when, because of high mortality rates, the average duration of a marriage was less than twenty years. Because so many were widowed, and about 10 per cent of the British population at this time did not marry at all, only about one-third of the population was married at any one time. [12]

But though there was at this time a strong delineation between the worlds inhabited by the married and the single, as in the first half of this century, there was also an in-between stage, one that continued virtually unaltered until the rules about marriage changed radically in the latter half of the eighteenth century. Formal marriage in church was, until then, but the final step in a complex process that had little to do with the Church or religious authority.

The *betrothal* of a man and a woman was almost more important than the actual marriage rite. It was far more than a mere promise to marry, or engagement. It was, rather, a public commitment between a man and a woman that, while not as binding as a marriage, was nevertheless solemnly observed. It did not always find favor with the Church, which had no part in it but could not dismiss it. At the heart of the betrothal rite, which differed in its detail from one locality to another, the couple made vows of consent to each other. Because the twelfth-century canon law of the Western Church recognized mutual consent as the basis for holy matrimony, church courts had to accept evidence of such commitment as a form of valid marriage.[13]

The time between betrothal and marriage was frequently seen as a time of permitted intimacy for the couple, even of sexual licence. It was not uncommon for couples to consummate their relationship after the betrothal ceremony.[14] It gave the protection of a public commitment to both parties, and

9

particularly to the woman, in case she became pregnant. In fact, there was, at many times and places, a high degree of pre-bridal pregnancy, varying from 10 per cent to 30 per cent of brides. In medieval times, couples often brought their child or children to a nuptial mass as a form of legitimizing them. In some parts of Britain, particularly during the early part of the Industrial Revolution, it was common for an engaged couple to marry only if the woman first "proved" her fertility by becoming pregnant. If she did not, the couple parted without shame, and each person took other suitors.[15]

In 1753, in response to the upper classes' concern about the ease of clandestine marriages which effectively removed the opportunity for parental control over unions, the British Government enacted the *Hardwicke Marriage Act*. This law terminated all the old rights both of clandestine unions and of betrothal, substituting instead the strict requirement that a marriage could take place only after the public reading of the banns over a three-week period, unless the couple purchased a licence from the bishop or his deputy. Parental consent for couples under twenty-one years of age was also strictly enforced.

The Act met with vigorous opposition before it was passed. Some opponents declared that it would "alter the very fabric of British society" and that in particular it would be very hard on women. They would lose the protection offered them by the old betrothal rites. Itinerant workers and others would find the residency requirements harsh, and many poor people would detest the formal public exposure that was an inevitable consequence of the reading of the banns. Unlike for the rich, however, the alternative of the private licence was not an option for them because of its expense.

Poorer people had no choice but to submit to the residential and other obligations of the "reading of the banns," with their highly unpopular corollary of publicity. The result was that among these people, common-law unions, although lacking the benefit and protection of the old betrothal rite, increased markedly over the next century. Illegitimacy also rose at an unprecedented rate. For the poor, however, illegitimacy was not as serious a stigma at this time as what it was later to become, when middle- and upper-class values began to dominate all sections of society. Premarital, and indeed marital, chastity had originally been the accepted standard only of the upper classes who had property to lose by any misalliance.[16]

Even into the early nineteenth century, working-class people still usually began sexual intimacy once a promise of marriage had been given, though rarely before. The promise was important, because women were reluctant to enter a full sexual relationship without some protection, because of their fear of pregnancy. It has been estimated that, in the period from the mid-eighteenth century to the mid-nineteenth century, as much as one-fifth of British people lived in a de facto relationship at some stage of their lives, usually as a prelude to marriage. Among the working classes, little shame was attached to premarital pregnancy, though increasingly in the middle classes women were expected to conform rigorously to the code of chastity on pain of loss of respectability.[17]

Indeed, there were some working-class women in Victorian Britain who reckoned that they were better off in common-law unions rather than in formal marriages. At a time when, on formal marriage, a woman lost all rights over her property, her children and even her legal identity, a common-law wife was still her own person. She retained her full rights over both her property and her children, and could seek the protection of the law against a violent "husband," which a married woman could not do. She was even able to seek maintenance for her children if her union broke up.[18]

The situation for unmarried mothers and de facto couples at this time was not dissimilar to what it is today, when recent changes to the law have extended access to government benefits and protection to sole parents and common-law partners not available earlier this century. Gillis argues that one factor in enforcing a more rigid pattern of expectation in the intervening period was the strict requirements on the part of the authorities in providing benefits for the dependents of fighting men during the First World War. Women had to prove legal marriage, and the legitimacy of their children, in order to receive dependency payments.[19]

From the second half of the nineteenth century, there occurred what Gillis has described as a "mass return to legal marriage," with common-law marriage retreating. Illegitimacy rates declined as well, and would not reach the early-nineteenth-century level until the 1960s. By the 1950s, British people were marrying at an earlier age, and more frequently, than at any other time in their history. The proportion of single people in the population dropped dramatically, as "monogamous marriage became virtually mandatory."[20]

How can we account for this enormous change? Certainly the power of rigorous Evangelical teaching over this period, with its focus on a narrow standard of personal morality, must be a factor. Combined with medical campaigns against venereal disease, a major cause of insanity in the days before antibiotics, it contributed to fears about all forms of extramarital sexuality, fears which became extreme, and often morbid. Strong Victorian notions of "respectability" also contributed to a situation that saw many otherwise healthy, normal people excessively fearful of anything to do with sex. The literature is full of examples of the immense damage such repression caused, even within marital relationships.

By the middle of the twentieth century, this pattern of rigidly narrow community expectations of sexual behaviour had reached its peak. It will be the task of future historians to evaluate fully just how and why this pattern disintegrated so quickly within the succeeding decades. It could be argued that it was principally the availability of reliable and acceptable forms of contraception in the 1960s that dramatically changed that pattern. In a matter of just a few short years, societal expectations of heterosexual conjugality reverted not just to previous patterns, but developed to a quite new stage of fluidity, without any historical precedent. "The Pill" allowed common-law relationships to flourish without any need of public betrothal rites or other forms of ceremonial acceptance that had once protected vulnerable women and their families against the worst consequences of unplanned pregnancy.

At the same time, the pattern of marriage practice has also reverted to one in which the Church plays an increasingly peripheral part. Since the 1970s, the numbers of people married in church have declined markedly. In 1973, when the Australian Federal Government licensed private marriage celebrants for the first time, 83.6 per cent of marriages were performed using some kind of religious rite. By 1993, this had fallen to 57.9 per cent, a decline of more than one-quarter. The decline occurred most rapidly in the decade up to 1983, when 60.6 per cent of marriage ceremonies were religious. Clearly this change is directly linked to the availability of attractive alternative forms of marriage ceremony, instead of the earlier sterile and restricted provision of a civil ceremony in the Registry Office. But that the government recognized and heeded the public need for an attractive alternative reflects a rapidly changing situation. The Church, for good or ill, represented conformity to a pattern of married life and sexuality rapidly being rejected by large sections of society. The slowdown in the growth of civil marriages in recent years might reflect the more realistic and generous views now held by most clergy, without there being a corresponding change in their churches' hierarchical pronouncements. As already mentioned, few clergy now quibble when couples present for marriage using a common address.[21]

The Church's role in this historical saga has by no means been uniform. In fact, it played little part in marriages in the first thousand years of Western Christianity. In the twelfth century, it made a concerted effort to regulate marriage, but mainly to ensure that the couple was not violating the Church's incest provisions and that both partners were freely consenting to the union. In canon law, after all, the requirement for a valid marriage was simply free and deliberate consent, not necessarily consent witnessed or mediated by a priest.

The major part of the complex public wedding rites in the medieval period actually took place away from the church building; the small rite that was conducted at the church was in the church porch. Medieval clergy, however, often took part with gusto in all the auxiliary community rites! It was not until the sixteenth century that the church was more fully involved at a formal level, with the marriage vows and consents exchanged inside the building. Even so, the service at the altar was still insignificant compared with the vast array of public festivities that accompanied the unions of all but the poorest of the poor. Church courts had a role in regulating sexual behavior, but they could only penalize a couple found cohabiting before marriage if there was no evidence of prior mutual consent necessary for a valid marriage provided for in the popular secular betrothal rites.[22]

Even in the period of the greatest controversy over marriage practices – the period from the *Hardwicke Marriage Act* of 1753 to when society by and large adopted the uniform practices of the upper classes in the second half of the nineteenth century – the Church was not a major player. It was, says Gillis, an issue not so much of religion as of class, as middle- and upper-class values won out over the more popular practices of the past.[23] By 1837, civil and nonconformist marriage had also become an option anyway, giving people not disposed to public or Anglican ceremonies a different means of formal marriage. For the first time, members of most of the Free Churches in England no longer had to submit to Anglican marriage rites.[24]

Nor was the Church always aware of the high number of people who were "married but not churched." Gillis cites incidences of nineteenth-century clerical ignorance of the many couples whose status in this regard was at least ambiguous. That, he says, indicate the enormous gulf that had developed between the educated, middle-class clergy and the bulk of the English population at that time.[25] It was only from the mid-eighteenth century that the Church has had, in British culture at least, a systematic level of control over marriage practice. Among the ordinary members of society, its views were often quite peripheral at times.

That is not to say that the Church did not have strong doctrinal views on marriage and sexuality throughout the historical period, but they were not *the same* views over that time. Just as patterns of marriage and sexual activity have changed, and changed often, so too the Christian Church has changed or adapted its doctrines and moral codes again and again, usually to meet the needs of the times though sometimes to meet its own needs of power and control. Historically, Christian moral standards have been surprisingly flexible. To a survey of these changing views we now turn.

2

NO SEX, PLEASE –
WE'RE CHRISTIANS!

Far from promulgating one clear, eternal teaching on sexuality, the Christian Church has in fact a checkered history of ambiguity on this subject. This is hardly surprising, as ambiguity is found within Christianity's most sacred text, the Bible. It is perhaps most evident in the attitudes displayed towards women, always a useful gauge of attitudes towards sexuality, as well as in the responses to marriage.

In the very first book of the Bible, Genesis, there are contradictory notions about the role of women. Indeed in the first chapter we are offered a vision of male–female equality when we are told God created both men and women in God's own image (Genesis 1: 27). However, in the second account of creation, in the second chapter, we learn that the woman is a secondary creation to the man, created specifically to be a "help meet" to him (Genesis 2:18–25).

In the New Testament, the same ambiguity can be traced. In his letter to the church at Galatia, the apostle Paul writes that in Christ there is neither male nor female (Galatians 3:28), but in other letters he argues that wives are subject to their husbands (Ephesians 5:22–24) and that women should cover their heads when they pray, as they are only the reflection of men, while men are no less than the "image and reflection of God" (1 Corinthians 11:6–7). While modern scholars might seek to explain or reconcile these differences and so give Paul a better press, the fact remains that these and other passages have had a profound effect throughout history on the way in which the Church has viewed both women and sexuality.

Ambivalences about marriage can also be found in the Scriptures. St Paul compares marriage with the relationship between Christ and his Church on the one hand (Ephesians 5:31–32) but, on the other, seems to express a clear preference for virginity (1 Corinthians 7:7, 32–34, 38). Again, while modern scholarship can provide a synthesis of these views, it is nevertheless true that, historically, these writings have been applied to detract from marriage, as we shall see.[1]

Building on these ambiguities, the Christian Church developed early an antithesis towards both women and marriage. Much has been written in recent times on the Church's views of women. While there would be little point in arguing the case afresh here, it is worth recalling that a consistently low view of women almost always prejudges views on marriage. Some writers have made the point that celibacy for the clergy implies not so much refraining from sexual activity as refraining from the company of women.[2] This conforms to the Church's long-held views that women are not only mentally and physically inferior to men, but spiritually inferior as well, and therefore constitute a danger to male spiritual welfare. It is tempting to imagine that such views have long been superseded, but the recent debates about women's ordination in the various branches of the Christian Church have established that views of female spiritual inferiority and danger continue unabated in some quarters, though they are rarely these days made explicit.[3]

Women were declared to be incomplete males by Aristotle – a view promoted by Christian theologians, and in particular by the influential thirteenth-century theologian Thomas Aquinas, who interpreted patristic theology from the standpoint of Aristotle's philosophy. A male child, on this view, was conceived in a perfect act of conception; a female – a deformed male – in an imperfect act. Further, the male seed carried all life; the female was but the incubator for the child "planted" by the male. The woman's primary sexual organ, the uterus, was believed directly to weaken the rationality of her mind, to make her hysterical, foolish, garrulous, deceitful, fearful, covetous, and feeble. These views of woman's inherent physical and mental inferiority, and of her subsidiary biological role, were not seriously challenged until developments in medical science in the last few centuries proved them incorrect.[4]

More important, however, is the view of women as morally and spiritually inferior to men, and more seriously, as the source of sin. This notion was derived from the Genesis story of the temptation of Adam and Eve, and was perhaps most fully expressed by the second-century theologian Tertullian. All women, he said, were Eve; all of them were "the devil's gateway," who brought sin into the world, tempted men to sin, and caused the Son of God to die.[5] A powerful indictment indeed.

Because women were believed to inflame men's passions against the male will, they were consistently required by the early Church fathers to refrain from all adornment, and to veil themselves in church. Because of the threat they posed, they were carefully segregated from men in worship, as they were in many other aspects of their lives. They were fully respected only if they remained virgins or at least renounced sexual activity after marriage; in other words, the only women fully accepted were women who denied their sexuality. Thus they were treated as honorary males, the only way in which they could redeem their secondary status. On and off throughout Christian history, there has even been a debate about whether women actually have souls or not. As late as 1588, there is a recorded case of an English clergyman in Essex seriously defending the proposition that women did not have souls.[6]

Fundamental to this distrust of women was a belief that their sexuality was intrinsically evil. The ancient fear of menstrual blood has made it a powerful taboo in many cultures, not least the Jewish culture, from which Christianity first sprang. As we shall see, there is a strong historical link between menstrual "impurity" and the call for celibacy. However, the fear ran even to childbirth itself which, it was believed, was defiling because of the flow of blood.

Leviticus 12:2–5 lays down rules for the purification of women following childbirth, and it is interesting to note that, for the Jews, giving birth to a female child rendered a woman doubly impure! After the birth of a son, a woman was impure for one week plus thirty-three days, during which time she was not allowed to touch any hallowed thing. If she gave birth to a daughter, her defilement lasted for two weeks plus sixty-six days! At the end of that time, she came to the priest, who made atonement for her, as if for sin, and thus restored her purity. So even the Virgin Mary had to go to the Temple in Jerusalem to be purified after the birth of the Son of God (Luke 2:22–23).

From about the eleventh century, the Christian Church has had services for the purification of women after childbirth. The first Anglican Prayer Book of 1549 called the service, adapted from a medieval rite, the "Purification of Women." Like the Old Testament rite, the Book of Common Prayer expected that the woman would undergo the service before touching any hallowed thing, or first receiving Communion after childbirth. She was also expected to wear a special white veil for the ceremony – a subject of much controversy during the Reformation, as the veil was the sign of penance and even of prostitution. However, until very recently, many English churches kept just such a veil ready for the occasion, and until the 1950s an astonishing number of English women still were "churched" after childbirth.[7]

By the second Prayer Book of 1552, the name had changed to a "Thanksgiving of women after childbirth, commonly called the churching of women." Though the name changed, in popular mythology it remained a ceremony of purification, and women were regarded as defiled until they had been "churched." It was the necessary gateway for their return to the community of the Church and, indeed, of society. Some held that a woman who died unchurched was automatically damned, and could not be buried in consecrated ground. Lesser old wives' tales had it that grass would wither if an unchurched woman walked on it. If the supreme female act of creation – ironically regarded by most women as a sacred experience – could be regarded as

19

intrinsically defiling and spiritually dangerous until very recent times, how much more was female sexuality believed to be dangerous during earlier centuries!

It is not surprising that the only truly acceptable woman was a virgin, a woman who effectively denied her sexuality completely. The Virgin Mary became the supreme exemplar, and over time was exalted to an unattainable position of reverence by virtue of her virginal sinlessness. Though it cannot be sustained from the biblical account, a whole theology of Mary as perpetual virgin developed. Part and parcel of this belief was a claim that Mary's physical virginity had remained intact despite the birth of Jesus. For Jesus had been born in a miraculous fashion, without any pain or even labor, leaving Mary's hymen intact and, significantly, uncontaminated by any flow of blood.[8] (Why she should then have needed purification in the Temple is not, however, explained.)

Mary as the image of the pure virgin and the model for all womanhood was celebrated from the earliest Christian centuries. The Church Fathers saw the image of the virgin body as a symbol of wholeness, and therefore holiness. By remaining virginal, a woman could escape the worst consequences of the Fall – the curse of childbirth, and rule by her husband. But she could even avoid that far graver symbol of corrupt flesh – menstruation – by fasting. In the early Christian centuries, young girls were urged to fast, and fast often. Strict fasting in young women can quickly result in the cessation of menstruation, at least temporarily, as is now well known in our society with the prevalence of anorexia nervosa. If the starvation is prolonged, menstruation can cease permanently. For St Jerome, for example, the feminine ideal was "women pale and thin with fasting."[9] Such women, of course, would not be sexually attractive – an important factor. Fasting, moreover, was often prescribed both for men and women as a means of reducing their sexual appetites.

The ahistorical image of the Virgin Mary was an impossible role model for flesh-and-blood women. No other woman could be both virgin and mother at the same time. So every woman who married and gave birth automatically fell short of spiritual perfection in a way that was not true for a man, merely by virtue of his being a husband or father. Even the most devout mother was in fact too close for comfort to the mirror-image stereotype: the scarlet woman, the whore. She too had a biblical image, in the persistent but incorrect labeling of Mary of Magdala as a fallen woman. It could be said that, historically, Christianity has had but two models of womanhood, that of virgin and whore. Effectively most women, then, have been left stranded between the two models, in uncomfortable ambiguity.

It is surely not coincidental that the greatest flowering of Marian devotion occurred during the early medieval period, as the Church began to enforce its long-held preference for celibacy of the clergy. As male theologians became increasingly divorced from the reality of women's lives, the image of the spotless asexual Mother of God assumed an unprecedented dominance. To say the least, it suggests to modern understanding an unhealthy psychosexuality.

The only truly acceptable woman was a virgin who consciously rejected her sexuality, even to the extent of punishing her body so that it was no longer fertile. Thus she became an honorary man. As Jerome put it:

> As long as a woman is for birth and children, she is different from man as body is from soul. But when she wishes to serve Christ more than the world [that is, by remaining virginal], then she will cease to be a woman, and will be called a man.[10]

Linked to the Early Church's attitude to women was a parallel attitude to the human body in general. This was most clearly exemplified in the growth of the monastic movement. In the Church's first centuries, Christians were tested by persecution. Until the peace of Constantine in the early fourth century, many thousands of Christians died as martyrs to the faith. Many others suffered terrible torments at the hands of persecutors, but survived. These "confessors," like the martyrs, were highly revered, and in the literature, at least, martyrdom was often longed for as offering entrance into heaven.

The centuries of persecution meant that the struggle for Christian perfection was characterized by suffering, even torment. When persecution ceased, the powerful imagery of the past could not easily be swept away. Instead, it was transferred from external persecution to self-inflicted punishment. Asceticism in every form became the watchword of the Church's teaching, as later Christians strove to outdo each other in self-denial.

The monastic movement was the most obvious aspect of this, and had an enormous impact on the rest of the Church. For the first monks, who lived in the desert of Egypt in the last decades of the third century, asceticism was rigorous. Perfection would only be attained by relentless self-mortification. Hard labour over long hours, little sleep and fasting would in time subdue the demands of the body and therefore of the soul, so that finally the ascetic might learn "over the long years of life in the desert, to do nothing less than to untwist the very sinews of his private will."[11] Significantly, the monk believed that his will had finally been subdued when he gained total mastery over his sexual fantasies. As long as his nights were disturbed by erotic dreams and nocturnal emissions, he knew he had not yet achieved the desired level of spiritual perfection, for his unruly sexuality was the supreme symbol of his "closed heart." This fear is echoed in a verse of the traditional Compline hymn, dating before the eighth century, which is still in regular use:

> From all ill dreams defend our eyes,
> From nightly fears and fantasies;
> Tread under foot our ghostly foe,
> That no pollution we may know.

Once sexual fantasies and experiences ceased, the monk believed it was proof that asceticism had been finally victorious.[12]

The monastic ascetic ideal spread, and was increasingly emulated by non-monastic clergy and laity. The result was that, by the fourth and fifth centuries, monastic literature was imbued with an almost hysterical fear and hatred of sex, and particularly of women, which far exceeded the more restrained attitudes of the monastic pioneers. There are stories of monks dipping their cloaks into the rotting flesh of a dead woman so that the smell would banish sensuous thoughts of her; of a young novice carrying his elderly mother across a stream with his hands fully covered by clothing, for fear that the flesh of all women is "fire." This has been identified as, in part, a misogyny contrived to protect the prestigious separation of the monks from the wider world. In turn, it strongly influenced the growing demand for clerical celibacy, another manifestation of prestigious separation from other Christians.[13]

These dominant attitudes to women and sex in the Church's early centuries could not but influence the approach to marriage that the Church Fathers adopted. The reluctant allowance St Paul seemed to grant to marriage as a state of life for Christians in his first letter to the Corinthians was also a powerful determinant of the Church's attitude: "I wish that all were as I myself am ... to the unmarried ... I say that it is well for them to remain unmarried as I am" (1 Corinthians 7:7–8). Paul's section on marriage in this letter was perhaps the most important of all influences on the Church's attitude to marriage, both before the sixteenth-century Reformation and within it. It was even taken up by the Protestant reformers, who turned it to their own advantage, as we shall see.

Building on St Paul, the early Church Fathers disseminated at best a reluctance about marriage, at worst a loathing for it, thus setting the Church on a similar course. The most influential of them was St Augustine of Hippo, whose treatise entitled *The Good of Marriage* set the pattern for later generations. There has been much controversy over this fifth-century writing. Scholars have argued over both its meaning and the extent to which it either genuinely praises or debunks marriage. But it is worth recalling that the treatise was written specifically to refute the claims of a "heretic" named Jovinian, who maintained that the married state

23

was equal in merit to virginity. Not so, responded Augustine, making it perfectly clear that virginity was vastly superior to marriage, and was indeed the more excellent way. "In no way can it be doubted that the chastity of continence is better than the chastity of marriage," he wrote.[14]

Because this treatise was so pivotal an influence on all later Christian theologies of marriage, it is worth exploring briefly the main arguments Augustine produced for his claims. Central to his thesis was the belief that sexual desire and the physical attributes of sexual performance were the direct result of original sin, the taint of which was passed through the human generations by the very act of procreation. Before the Fall, intercourse would have been performed calmly, rationally, without "lascivious heat or unseemly passion," he maintained. But the lust necessary even for procreative acts since the Fall reveals, for Augustine, its sinful corruption.

Augustine's equation of purity with self-control and rationality is not unique. He was merely reflecting the ascendancy which Hellenistic dualism had gained in Christian thought during its first centuries, despite its struggles against dualistic heresy in other directions. One of the chief features of this thought was the abhorrence of emotion and feeling; renunciation and ascetical discipline were the means to spiritual victory over sin. The physical and emotional abandon necessary in sexual intercourse was dangerous, and tainted with evil. Augustine, however, like other early Christian leaders, could not denounce marriage outright, for all his preference (in theory at least) for total sexual abstinence. In the biblical record, marriage had, after all, been instituted by God in the Garden of Eden; Christ had affirmed it, and even turned a country wedding into a never-to-be-forgotten feast. The Church Fathers could not, then, denounce marriage as completely evil as did the dualist heresies of the time. The "convenient distinction between the good and the better" provided the answer, and Augustine excelled in capitalising on that distinction. *The Good of Marriage*, for all that it attempts to ascribe a severely restricted "goodness" to the married state, is nevertheless based on the premise that virginity is always and everywhere the "better" state.

In defining marriage as "good," Augustine attributes to it three "goods" which were to permeate all subsequent Christian marriage theology — offspring, fidelity, and sacrament. "Procreation" is the first and primary reason for marriage, and the only acceptable reason for sexual intercourse. Within marriage the gratification of sexual desire other than for the express purpose of conceiving a child is not sinless, though because of the marriage it is pardoned. It is, in other words, a "venial" sin. (If the married couple actually derives pleasure from the sexual act it swiftly becomes a mortal sin, however!) "Fidelity," to Augustine, means more than simply sexual faithfulness to the marriage partner; it also encompasses the legalistic concept of the obligation of one partner to meet the sexual need of the other — the marriage "debt." In this artificial scenario, the partner who acquiesces to the need of the other is guiltless of any sin, but the one who asks for satisfaction is guilty. "Sacrament," for Augustine, did not convey the sacramental understanding as it would develop much later in the Church. Rather, it refers to the indissoluble nature of Christian marriage. Though the mutual companionship or love between a husband and wife is praised by Augustine, it is by no means central, and has no place within the three essential "goods."[15]

From this view of sexual intercourse espoused by Augustine, it is easy to see where the Church derived its long-standing absolute prohibition on any form of contraception other than abstinence. If the only truly acceptable reason for sexual intercourse is for the express procreation of children, then clearly contraception is forbidden, as made plain in the 1968 Papal encyclical *Humane Vitae*, still in force in the Roman Catholic Church. It is worth remembering, however, that even the Reformed churches stood firm against all forms of contraception until relatively recent times, arguing from a similar standpoint. These churches changed their minds and overturned one of Christianity's most enduring prohibitions, a point to which we will return.[16]

Even though procreation is the one "good" that gives marriage its *raison d'être*, Augustine nevertheless makes it plain that even the generation of children is not a supreme ideal. Continence is better than marital intercourse even for the sole purpose of procreation, because the City of God would be more quickly filled and the end of time hastened if all people would only restrain themselves from all sexual activity. Marriage – and here we can hear the voice of St Paul (1 Corinthians 7:9) – is only for those who cannot control themselves, and even they should strive to reach a "higher grade of sanctity" by denying their impulses.

For Augustine, the most chaste of marriages falls short of the perfection of chastity available to those who totally abstain from sexual activity. Marriage, at its best, is merely a concession to the weak. Though Augustine gave these views a cohesion and status that was to make them extremely influential during the following millennium and beyond, he was certainly not their inventor. They can be traced back through the first Christian centuries to St Paul himself, and are in a sense the culmination of the anti-women, anti-marriage and anti-sexuality theories that had developed over those years.

Part of this developing theology was, not suprisingly, the growing demand for a celibate, or at least sexually inactive, priesthood. It is interesting to note that the original New Testament ministerial ideal, expressed in the pastoral epistles, was that clergy should be exemplary married men, who had proved that they could rule the Church by their ability to raise good children and govern their households well (1 Timothy 3:2–4, 12, and Titus 1:6). This expectation, however, could not survive the increasing patristic exaltation of asceticism, and particularly of virginity. By the third century, one Church Father, Origen – who so loathed sexual activity that he allegedly castrated himself – was urging the ideal of a celibate priesthood.[17]

The first express demand that the clergy be sexually continent came out of a local synod, held in Elvira, Spain, in the first decade of the fourth century. Among a large number of canonical regulations designed to control rigidly all Christian sexual behavior is Canon 33, which required all clergy to abstain totally from their wives, and not to beget children. It was not *celibacy* (non-marriage) that was required, but abstention from sex within marriage. This prohibition, then, was not a requirement for clergy to live the single life for the better service of the Lord. Rather, it was a prohibition made simply in the interests of cultic purity, as there is no suggestion in the canons that the clergy should not remain as married men.[18]

The wording of Canon 33 and of the other canons dealing with sexuality reveals an implicit assumption that sexual activity *per se* was dangerous and defiling and constituted a threat to Christian identity. It reflects a natural, even an inevitable, progression from the growing cultic and sacral emphasis evident in Christian ministry in the preceding century. The canons of Elvira, taken together, single out the clergy from the laity in the promotion of a clerical élite based on sexual asceticism. Those who live pure, sacrificial lives that mark them off from even the strictly controlled laity deserve leadership status. They reveal the "close connection in the ancient church between clerical taboos against sexuality and the formation of a clerical elite."[19]

The Elvira Canon was the product of only a local church council, but it was the beginning of a process that would quickly gain momentum. At the Council of Nicaea in 325, Bishop Ossius of Cordova, a member of the Elvira Synod, proposed universal adoption of the canon. However, according to a later account, his attempt was thwarted by a stand, taken supposedly in support of marriage by an Egyptian monk, Paphnutius, revered as a "confessor of the faith" for his acute sufferings under persecution. Paphnutius, though obviously unmarried himself, declared that sexual intercourse within marriage was chaste according to early church historians. The sixteenth-century reformers would later make much of his statement.

Conveniently, they would ignore the second part of Paphnutius' reported speech, which reminded the Council of the Church's ancient tradition which, while allowing married men to be ordained, prevented men from marrying at all once ordained.[20]

The first attempt to impose clerical chastity as a universal law came some sixty years later, in the first authentic papal decretal of 385. Pope Siricius commanded continence for reasons clearly linked to the need for cultic purity for the Eucharistic celebration. He compared the Christian priesthood with the Jewish Levitical priests who, he claimed, had been commanded to dwell apart from their wives for a year at the time of their service in the Temple. This was so that, "adorned with a pure conscience, they might offer to God an acceptable sacrifice." How much more, then, should Christian priests, from the time of their ordination, keep their "bodies in soberness and modesty, so that in those sacrifices which we offer daily to our God we may please him in all things"?[21]

It is not coincidental that demands for permanent cultic purity came at the same time that the practice of daily celebration of the Eucharist was gaining ground. In the fourth century, continence was expected of all Christians before taking the sacrament, so as daily masses became commonplace in the Western Church the requirement of permanent continence for the clergy was a logical extension. In the Eastern Church, where there was no daily celebration, a fully married priesthood remained possible.[22]

The notion that the Christian priesthood was directly descended from the Aaronic priesthood arose in the third century, and was to have a significant impact on the growing demand for clerical chastity. Pope Siricius' successors repeated his claims about the cultic separation of the Old Testament priests from their wives, but in fact the only evidence that there was any separation comes from the Mishnah, which states the High Priest was removed from his house seven days before he offered the sacrifice on the Day of Atonement. A rabbinic commentary claims that this was to ensure that the priest did not render himself cultically impure through contact with menstrual blood. The fear was not of sexual intercourse at all. Some have suggested the possibility that the ancient taboo against menstrual blood lies behind the celibacy law and, indeed, behind the prohibition of women priests.[23]

So by the end of the fourth century, the die was cast in no uncertain terms. The Christian Church's first consistent, formalized standard of sexual behavior was uncompromising. Indeed, it might be said to offer clear "certainty." All sexual activity, even within marriage, even for nothing but the express purpose of procreation, was defined as inherently defiling and, even worse, potentially mortally dangerous to the Christian soul. The only completely acceptable lifestyle for Christians that protected them against this danger was absolute sexual abstinence. Human sexuality was not for one moment seen as a good gift of God; in fact it was the exact opposite: a punishment the human race repeatedly paid for the Fall. Marriage was no more than the necessary but distasteful means of propagating the human race – again a penalty of the Fall – and a concession to the weakness instilled in humans through their primal disobedience.

The demand for a sexually chaste priesthood for reasons of cultic purity demonstrated and promoted this standard powerfully. Christian people could have been in no doubt at all on the subject. That these demands quickly and effectively established a special, élite clerical caste that the humble laity could in no way emulate is no accident. Again and again, the Church has used moral and other codes of behavior in order to impose authority and gain power for certain privileged groups. The temptation is not very far away today.

This sexual standard reigned supreme in the Church for the best part of 1500 years. It was not, however, a particularly easy standard to enforce! Until the eleventh and twelfth centuries, there was no powerful central control to assist the ecclesiastical authorities. The papacy, while holding a spiritual preeminence, had little power over the diverse dioceses of the Western Church. So from when the first demands were issued that married clergy live with their wives "like sisters," church officials had their work cut out finding ways of enforcing those demands.

The first to submit were, not surprisingly, the higher clergy: generally ambitious men who had too much to lose by failing to conform. Married bishops were the first to feel disfavor if their marriages were not obviously asexual. Monk-bishops in sixth-century Gaul turned up the heat on their married brothers, and frequently attacked the bishops' wives as evil, lustful, and hindrances to their husbands.

The records of this period reveal the myriad regulations that became necessary to police the abstinence required in clerical marriages. In Gaul, a trial year of continence was introduced before a man was raised to the diaconate; his wife's permission was necessary for his ordination. Those clerics who did return to conjugal relations were often accused of committing a form of incest. Further regulations stipulated that husband and wife must not share the same bed or the same room, and bishops in particular were to live surrounded by their clergy in order to avoid any suspicion of marital intimacy. [24]

This ludicrous situation of a married but supposedly continent clergy continued until the eleventh century. For centuries, the clergy struggled with a clash between the reality and an impossible ideal. Given the hysterical fear that women posed unimaginable threats to male sanctity, it is surprising that the permission for clergy to remain married survived the first centuries of Christianity at all. Perhaps the married-but-continent rule began as a political compromise that at least established an ideal that effectively set the clergy apart.

The rule was not popular, however; it was unenforceable, and demonstrably unworkable. Before the reforming Gregorian popes began to centralize power in Rome, most priests – certainly those in rural areas – were married men for whom the ideal of chaste marital relations was, not surprisingly, rarely achieved. And despite the long-standing theoretical rule prohibiting marriage after ordination, the marriage of priests already ordained was still regarded as valid, though illicit.

Ascetics like Peter Damian, the eleventh-century Benedictine monk and Doctor of the Church, renowned for his uncompromising teachings on personal austerity and mortification, believed the limited concession of marriage was destroying the clerical ideal, and worse, was encouraging gross immorality among the clergy. The ready availability of wives to the lower clergy was simply too great a temptation, and incited sins even worse than marital sexual activity. Removal of the temptation would remove the sin.[25]

The Gregorian "reforms" were based on this argument. Three decrees of Gregory VII — issued in 1059, 1063, and 1074 — ordered that the faithful laity were not to attend the masses conducted by clergy known to have intimate relations with women. A decree of 1123 barred all higher clergy from marriage. However, the critical decree was that promulgated by the Second Lateran Council of 1139, which declared clerical marriage actually invalid for the first time. The permission for a married man to be ordained, provided he took a vow of continency, remained in force technically, but fell rapidly into disuse. During this period of reform, the distinction between clergy wives and concubines became blurred, thus heightening connotations of immorality even in valid pre-ordination marriages.[26]

Despite isolated episodes of agitation for a relaxation of obligatory celibacy in both the fourteenth and fifteenth centuries, and strong attempts at the Council of Trent to conciliate the German Protestants by allowing a married clergy, the law remained, and remains, in force for the Roman Catholic Church. Indeed, in 1563 the Council of Trent declared those who promoted clerical marriage to be anathema (Canon 9).

The main point of dispute in the Trent debate seemed to be over the origin of the celibacy law, with a minority seeking to claim it as being of divine origin against the majority opinion that it was an ecclesiastical law. It was the continuing toleration of a married clergy in the Eastern Church that prevented the "divine law" proponents from making much ground. The Council of

Trent, in fact, succeeded in establishing a general observance of the celibacy law for the first time, through the seminary system that it inaugurated.[27]

What lay behind the Western Church's consistent opposition to clerical marriage from the fourth century onwards? The original interpretation was that virginity, as the higher lifestyle, was the only fitting one for the Christian priesthood. But most twentieth-century scholars have argued that the driving motive was cultic purity: "He who stands at the altar must keep himself away from the sexual act." Certainly this fits with the first papal demand for celibacy, which linked it to the supposed precedent of the cultic separation of the Old Testament priests, and it can be shown to have appeared consistently in other documentation over the centuries.[28]

Peter Damian expressed the cultic purity argument in its most extreme and elaborate form:

> If, therefore, our Redeemer so loved the bloom of perfect chastity that he was not only born of a virgin womb, but also fondly handled by a virgin foster-father, and this while he was still an infant crying in the cradle, by whom, I ask, does he wish his Body to be handled, now that he is reigning in all his immensity in heaven?[29]

The cultic purity argument – mainly in the form of the well-used comparison with the Old Testament priests' cultic obligations – was pressed again at the Council of Trent, and has been repeated frequently until very recent times. It was the argument that was used overwhelmingly against the sixteenth-century reformers' counter-arguments for a married clergy. Certainly, the fact that until the Gregorian reforms it was sexual activity and not marriage itself that was prohibited to the clergy indicates that these arguments were more than mere rhetoric. The belief that sexual intercourse – even in marriage – was somehow always defiling, and the consequent restrictions placed on lay marital sexuality in connection with presence at the Eucharist, indicate that cultic purity concerns operated quite separately from the question of clerical celibacy *per se*. The underlying fear and denial of women can be discerned in all these motives: only men who abstain from all women are pure enough to handle the Body and Blood of Christ, are sufficiently set apart from the laity to lead the Church, and are holy enough to maintain strict morality.

A moment's reflection indicates the enormity of this view. If married men in normal marital relations with their wives cannot handle the sacrament, if sexual intercourse even for the conceiving of children is always defiling, what does this say about human sexuality? Nothing less than that it is by its very nature sinful, and even evil. What it says about women is that they are, quite simply, beyond the pale, for any contact with them renders men, and particularly priests, impure.

The Elvira Canon, we noted, in one sense established a clerical élite by its demands of total sexual abstinence for the clergy. That is one aspect of clerical celibacy that has no doubt persisted. But motives other than those connected with cultic purity – motives both implicit and explicit – can be discerned.

On practical grounds, the eleventh- and twelfth-century reforming popes were keen to stamp out the inheritance of benefices by priests' sons and the subsequent hereditary succession that effectively weakened hierarchical control of the local church. Pope Gregory VII most frequently required celibacy out of obedience to papal power.[30] He and his fellow reforming popes were bent on creating a cohesive, powerful church exercising supreme control over all its bishops and priests, undistracted by competing loyalties to family or lineage. A body of celibate men bound only to the Church, and therefore easier to discipline and direct, was crucial to the power structure they sought.

This motivation was not necessarily confined to the Middle Ages. In more recent times, an Australian priest, Paul Collins, has written:

> Underlying Rome's insistence on celibacy is the question of power. The celibate man is the Church's

> man with no other focus to his life except the Church
> ... Economically, psychologically, and spiritually he is
> the Church's man, tied to it through a network of
> dependency.[31]

The Christian Church's traditional teaching on sex and marriage
was the product of celibate male theological reflection. The vast
majority of the priests who wrote on the subject were
themselves – as members of religious orders or high-ranking
clergy – unmarried. If they had any experience of sexual love, it
was covert, and therefore compromised, and bound to heighten
their sense of the sinfulness of sex, given the thought-world in
which they lived.

It would be helpful to know how much their strict rules and
attitudes affected the laity, who were after all the only people
expected to marry. But it is an impossible task to gain full access
to the responses of married men and women, even in the
medieval and early-modern periods. Laypeople left few records
of their theological views, and so the historian is hampered to a
large degree.

However, we can understand something of the way in which
the teaching percolated down to the laity, through the existing
confession manuals of the medieval clergy. These manuals are
powerfully imbued with the fear of sexual pleasure. Their clerical
writers "found the marital bed a dangerous place for people who
would remain faithful to the law."[32] The advice to confessors
strayed far from the common experience of married people
through hairsplitting discussions on the permissible motives for
sexual intercourse within marriage, and indeed questioned
married people even on the positions adopted. If in no other way,
lay people learned in the confessional the myriad dangers
attending sexual desire. And the rules governing marital sex were
not limited merely to the motives and positions for intercourse.
They also covered the times during which intercourse was
permitted. Traditionally, married people were not to indulge on
Wednesdays or Fridays (the Church's fast days), nor on Saturdays

(the eve of Sunday and therefore of the weekly Eucharist), nor on Sundays. The whole of Lent was out, along with other fast days, major feasts and their eves, and during the times when women were either menstruating (the old taboo again) or lactating. The linkage of forbidden sex to the cultic purity requirements of the Eucharist, and to times of penance, is no stronger than the linkage to the particular times of female "impurity." Taken together, there was not very much time for sexual activity at all!

The laity also learned of the expectations of the Church's teaching through popular literature. A particularly useful example is Geoffrey Chaucer's *The Parson's Tale*, from *The Canterbury Tales*. This work is little known to modern readers. Written in formal prose – in the form of a solemn treatise on penitence – instead of in Chaucer's distinctive dramatic style, it is omitted from most selections of the *Tales*, and is ignored by modern renderings. However, there is no reason to believe that it was not as widely read as the other tales in the fifteenth and sixteenth centuries, when Chaucer's work was in wide circulation.

The Parson's Tale, based on two influential thirteenth-century confession manuals, presents contemporary orthodox Christian doctrine, without any hint of innovation. Given Chaucer's depiction of the Parson himself as a model of true piety and an ideal parish priest, his *Tale* is clearly meant to present what was regarded as central doctrine.[33]

Not surprisingly, the *Tale* teaches that virginity is the perfect state, and most certainly so for the clergy. It goes on to depict the sinfulness and lechery that can exist within the marriage bond, and counsels husbands against loving their wives immoderately:

> Man shulde loven his wyf by discretion, paciently and atemprely [moderately] and thanne is she as though it were his suster. [34]

The Parson describes, as a species of adultery, the marriage act committed for pleasure:

> The thridde spece of avowtrie is sometyme betixe a
> man and his wyf, and that is whan they take no reward
> in hire assemblynge [union] but oonly to hire flesshly
> delit …[35]

The union of husband and wife merely for "amorous love" is "deadly sin," he expounds. The Parson also lays down the rules of the Christian home. Wives must obey their husbands in all things, be honest and discreet at all times, and most certainly should never have authority over their husbands.[36]

The very antithesis of the Parson's model wife was, however, a fellow pilgrim on the journey to Canterbury! The Wife of Bath is a celebrated character in English literature, and was by no means discreet or "mesurable." Nor is it likely that she ever obeyed *her* husbands. Her lively prologue is the counterbalance to almost the entire corpus of the Parson's teaching on sex and marriage, and suggests that the laity were probably little inclined to observe the Church's rigorous regulations, though they clearly knew them full well. Her prologue is in fact a spirited defense of marital sexuality. Even so, she is not ignorant of the Church's teachings, and her doctrinal knowledge seems sound. She recognizes the superiority of virginity and even of continent marriage, but cheekily claims St Paul's dictum as her justification for marrying again and again:

> Wedding's no sin, so far as I can learn.
> Better it is to marry than to burn.[37]

She obviously knew the Church's teaching that the marriage act should be employed only for either procreation or the "payment of the debt," but by shrewd manipulation of these rules, she makes it abundantly clear that she sees sex as primarily for pleasure:

> In wifehood I will use my instrument
> As freely as my Maker me it sent.
> If I turn difficult, God give me sorrow!

> Whenever he likes to come and pay his debt,
> I won't prevent him! I'll have a husband yet
> Who shall be both my debtor and my slave
> And bear his tribulation to the grave
> Upon his flesh, as long as I'm his wife.
> For mine shall be the power all his life
> Over his proper body, and not he,
> Thus the Apostle Paul has told it me,
> And bade our husbands they should love us well;
> There's a command on which I like to dwell …[38]

Although based on the same doctrines, the difference between the *Wife of Bath's Prologue* and *The Parson's Tale* could not be greater; indeed, the Wife's abundant sexual appetite fully bears out the Church's deep mistrust of women as temptresses of men! Chaucer's treatment of the Wife surely indicates that, whatever pious doctrine might have said, at least some lay people did not let it destroy their marital pleasures.

However, the Wife is not a particularly devout woman, for all that she is going on pilgrimage. For the more serious-minded and deeply pious married laity, the Church's teaching must have presented nothing short of a minefield for them to negotiate throughout their married lives. No wonder virginity, or at least continent marriage, seemed attractive.

For the best part of 1500 years, until the sixteenth century, the Christian Church's standards of sexual morality, and its attitudes to sex, were plain. Women were by their very nature impure, the cause of sin, and a constant danger to male sanctity. Male sexual desire, while never as evil as women's, was nevertheless also the preeminent sign of flawed humanity. Sexual activity, even within marriage – and for the express purpose of procreation only – was always defiling. Any other forms of marital sexuality were sinful, and were as grave a threat to the human soul as extramarital sexuality. Virginity, protected by fasting and other acts of self-mortification, was the only sure way of achieving Christian perfection, while sexual abstinence designed to ensure cultic purity at the altar was obligatory. Those who taught these precepts backed them up consistently with the evidence of Scripture and of the Fathers, and there was proof in plenty for them to find in both places. Those who seek the most consistently taught and long-standing Christian rules on sexuality need look no further. That such rules appal our modern consciousness should not deter those who demand moral absolutes and certainty.

These standards have imbued all Christian thought and teaching, all Western culture. Though no longer generally taught, their influence lingers still, deep in the psyche of twentieth-century men and women. They underlie much of modern society's sexual obsession and dysfunction. They reinforce attitudes that want eternally to separate the sacred and the secular, the soul and body, rationality and desire. A mere four hundred years or so of a process of changing the teaching of the ages has not yet been long enough to root out this terrifying legacy of Christian teaching.

But at the intellectual level at least, the Church did change its mind. Recognizing at least some of the limitations of the ancient code, and faced with a new set of problems, the sixteenth-century reformers began the long and as yet incomplete process of turning that code upside down.

3

SHIFTING
THE GROUNDRULES

Halfway through the second Christian millennium, the groundrules for sex in Christian doctrine began to change. The flowering of the Renaissance in Europe, with its fundamental shifts in understandings of human potential, achievement, and individuality, could not but affect views of sexuality. However, what we would understand as a modern theological approach to sex leaped fully formed neither from the Renaissance womb nor, for that matter, from the imagination of the Protestant reformers. It would take a century and more of heated debate before a recognizably modern attitude began to gain ground.

Its faint beginnings can be traced in literature from the second half of the fifteenth century. A distinguished French theologian, Martin Le Maistre (1432–1481), swept away all the hair-splitting Augustinian distinctions on the purposes of marital intercourse. Indeed, he went so far as to approve of married sex for the "calming of the mind," and even for pleasure. It was a dangerous doctrine, he said, to say that marital sex for pleasure was a mortal sin, for by that doctrine a man might as readily have intercourse with any woman as with his wife! He was followed by a Scots theologian, John Major (1470–1550), who maintained that it was no more sin for a husband and wife to copulate for pleasure than "to eat a handsome apple for the pleasure of it." To take an opposite view, he said, "was to convict many married people (as I guess) of sin." Neither Le Maistre nor Major managed to influence the mainstream orthodox theologians of their time, who condemned them; but the writings of the two men indicate that orthodoxy was being seriously challenged at last.[1]

A major challenge from quite a different direction came from one of the leading humanists of the immediate pre-Reformation period. John Colet (1466?–1519), an English priest and scholar, was an austere humanist who lived a life of intense personal piety and withdrawal from society. His views on sexuality are harsh, but in two important areas they provided an avenue for later developments. In the late fifteenth century, Colet lectured at Oxford University on the epistles of St Paul, and it was at this time that he developed his *Exposition* of the first letter to the Corinthians. His exegesis of chapter seven, the scriptural passage at the heart of the celibacy debate, provided the vehicle for his discussion of marriage.

Colet was in no doubt whatsoever that celibacy was the ideal for all people. As Christ was chaste, so all Christians should strive to be chaste too, as far as they are able:

> It is plainly evident, that all who wish to be Christians, must endeavour to resemble Christ to the utmost of their power; and must not stop short at any point, of their own free will, until they have attained to Him.[2]

However, unlike earlier theologians, Colet accepted that chastity was not possible for all people. Some were not able to reach that height of perfection, even though they longed for it. These people could marry, he said, and be pardoned for their failure. Marriage, for Colet, was a concession, or indulgence, to human weakness. And as such, its primary purpose was as a remedy for sin, "when by the mutual succour it affords, it keeps married men from roaming at large, and wantoning among women." Even so, marriage was not a license for sexual enjoyment, but a "remedy for involuntary desire, not a house of call for self-sought gratification."[3] In fact, Colet saw "remedy" as constituting the only reason for marriage. Not for him the traditional view that marriage's only valid purpose was procreation; for him there was, since Christ, no longer any need for prolonging human generation. If all were celibate, the "day of the Lord" would come so much more quickly.

Colet's teaching here represents a radical break with Christian orthodoxy, which had always taught that engaging in marital sex in order to avoid worse temptation was sinful. Though he seems to offer a distasteful and ultimately unrealistic reason for marriage, he nevertheless provided a theology of marriage that at least recognized the legitimacy of human sexual need, albeit in a crude and limited way. Most importantly, this recognition went so far as to allow that the ideal of celibacy was not possible for all people, because of the demands of their sexual needs. This argument, in time, paved the way for an acceptance that not all clergy could attain the perfection of chastity and so should marry, though Colet himself never argued the case for a married clergy directly. To the contrary, when he was Dean of St Paul's, London, he even required that the Cathedral Virger be celibate, as it was "fitting that those who approach so near to the altar of God, and are present at such great mysteries, should be wholly chaste and undefiled."[4] Nevertheless, his claim that celibacy was impossible for some was innovative, as orthodoxy had always maintained that all could achieve celibacy by prayer, fasting, and other forms of self-discipline. Colet's attitudes to sexuality are the epitome of the centuries of teachings offered by celibate theologians with no understanding of the reality of married experience.

By contrast, Colet's biographer Desiderius Erasmus offered a vision of marriage that is positive, warm, and attractive. Erasmus, one of the most influential figures in the prelude to the Protestant Reformation, lived for some years in England. In 1497 or 1498, he wrote his *Encomium Matrimonii*, an epistle in praise of marriage for his pupil William Mountjoy, to whom he was teaching rhetoric. Erasmus was later to claim that his work had clearly been more successful than as a mere text in the art of rhetoric, for by the time the work was first published in 1518 Mountjoy had already outlived three wives, and was perhaps considering marrying a fourth.[5]

In this work, Erasmus claimed it as his central proposition that the state of marriage was of a value equal to that of celibacy. He was rapidly criticized as a heretic for such a preposterous claim, a claim he nevertheless defended. Whether the pro-marriage views Erasmus enunciated in this work – designed after all to teach the art of rhetoric – were truly his own views is not certain.[6] However, they had wide currency in Europe at a time when all theological views were in the melting pot and could not help but be influential.

The *Encomium Matrimonii* presents marriage in a manner that is almost the mirror image of the theology offered by Colet in virtually the same year. Unlike his friend, Erasmus stood firm by the traditional view of marriage as primarily for procreation. He encouraged his pupil to marry to ensure the continuation of his family line, but also encouraged the growth of a larger population. The very survival of Christendom was at stake, he said, for want of a population large enough to provide sufficient fighting men to hold back the Turks. "Bachelorship," to Erasmus, equalled barrenness, which was against the Mosaic law. In fact, denial of marriage – and therefore of begetting children – came close to the crimes of abortion and contraception, he maintained.

But Erasmus went much further. The unmarried state was reviled as "unnatural." Marriage was ordained not only by the Creator, but by "Dame Nature" herself. It is the law of nature, "inwardly fixed in our hearts," and it "seemeth a foul shame dumb beasts to obey the laws of nature, and men ... to bid battle against nature." Even inanimate nature experiences a form of marriage, he writes, as the heaven moves above the earth with continual turning, and the earth, lying underneath, is made fruitful by the seed that the heaven pours on the earth like a husband. Indeed, the desire for marriage is so integral to all nature that not to desire marriage is unnatural.[7]

So Erasmus defines sexuality as essential to the very order of nature created by God, denial of which means rebellion against that order. He equates true manhood with willingness to accept the sexual role. He becomes even more explicit in his defense of the innate goodness of the human sex drive:

> Whereas all other things be ordained by nature with most high reason, it is not likely that she slumbered and slept in making only this prize member. For I hear him not which will say unto me that that foul itching and pricks of carnal lust have come not of nature, but of sin. What is more unlike the truth? As though matrimony (whose office cannot be executed without those pricks) was not before sin. Moreover to other beasts I pray you from whence cometh those pricks and provocations? Of nature; or of sin? Wonder it is if not of nature. And as touching the foulness, surely we make that by our imagination to be foul, which of the self nature is fair and holy ... But virtue (ye say) is to be obeyed rather than nature. As though that is to be called virtue which repugneth with nature ...[8]

Erasmus even goes so far as to commend married life for the pleasure of sexual activity, which within marriage gives no offense either to God or society. There is no place here for marriage as "remedy" for sin or "concession" to weakness. This is at many removes from the deep distaste and suspicion of sex, and particularly marital sexuality, evident in the writings of the Fathers, the medieval theologians, and even contemporaries such as Colet. Nearly a century later, Erasmus' views were still being attacked as "naturalist" and "Pelagian," which gives some idea of their innovation for their time.[9]

For all that, Erasmus does not give sexual intimacy in marriage a high rating. It is in fact not really very important, he maintains: "albeit the pleasure of bodies is the least part of the goods that wedlock has."[10] Rather, marriage's greatest joys, for Erasmus, lie in companionship and domesticity. These are the baits to lure a bachelor into marriage. A wife is one who loves without falsehood, who comforts a man in time of trouble, who drives away the "tediousness of solitary being." Marriage, says

Erasmus, was instituted by God primarily for companionship, because after God had created Adam he thought that his life "should be utterly miserable and unpleasant, if he joined not Eve a companion unto him." Contrary to the traditional Christian understanding that marriage survives only until "death do us part," Erasmus suggests married love is eternal. Such a concept could only strengthen marriage's intrinsic worth in comparison with the usual teaching that it was virginity that was of heavenly value.[11]

Parenthood has joys, too, beyond the fulfilling of duty to family and society. In a passage so touching and memorable that a later-sixteenth-century English writer, Thomas Becon, would use it (without acknowledgment) in his own praise of parenthood, Erasmus wrote:

> Now sir, how highly will ye esteem this thing, when your fair wife shall make you a father with a fair child? When some little young babe shall play in your hall which shall resemble you and your wife? Which with a mild lisping or amiable stammering, shall call you Dad?[12]

This warm, realistic and engaging depiction of domestic happiness is something that all the long centuries of sterile debate about marriage conducted by theologians and canonists had not even hinted at.

In fact, Erasmus rejects all the usual practical arguments against marriage, particularly that which depicts wives and children as nothing but trials. It is not the fault of marriage if they are trials, he insists. Rather, it is human error. Women's behavior is often governed by the way their husbands behave towards them, he says, and good men can reform evil wives. Good children are born of good parents. All people, he concludes, are subject to the chances of fortune: "He must get him out of the world which will here no incommodity."[13]

Erasmus offers a theological explanation for his high view of matrimony. It is, he says, the primary sacrament, the one ordained first. The others, he insists, were ordained on earth for the remedy of fallen human nature. But marriage was ordained in paradise, at the first creation, for human "solace." The novelty here is that Erasmus avoids any suggestion that marriage, at least since the Fall, is ordained also for the remedy of sin. Marriage belongs as much to the new law of Christ as to the old law of Moses, he writes in refutation of those who consign it solely to the earlier law.

If Christ regarded marriage so highly, why did he not himself marry?

> As though there be not very many things in Christ, which we ought rather to marvel at, than follow. He was born without carnal father, he proceeded without pain of his mother, he arose from death to live ... what is not in him above nature? ... Let us (living within the law of nature) wonder and praise the things that be above nature, but follow those works that be for our capacity.[14]

This passage is a powerful indicator of Erasmus' attitude to compulsory celibacy. Virginity, he confesses, is a "divine thing, an angelical thing." But marriage, for Erasmus, is "an human thing." He pays lip service to the orthodox notion that virginity is a higher state of life than marriage, but makes it clear that this is because virginity is a state that belongs to a realm other than the human. In other words, marriage, not virginity, is the state designed for humans to live in. Virginity is for the few, designed by God as a "certain token" of the heavenly life, in which marriage is no more. Marriage, he insists, is as holy a lifestyle:

> ... he is but a very little off from the praise of virginity, which keepeth purely the law of wedlock, and which hath a wife to the intent to beget children, and not to satisfy his wanton lust.[15]

It is interesting that here Erasmus reverts to a more conventional view of marital sexuality in his attempt to compare it to the holiness of virginity. Perhaps this reversion is because he wants to define marital sex as a lifestyle holier than that of the "swarms of monks, friars, canons," for Erasmus was strong in his call for clerical marriage. His main reason was developed in response to the public infamy attracted by the dissolute lifestyle of so many supposedly chaste priests:

> How much better were it to turn their [the priests'] concubines into wives, so that those whom they now have with great infamy, and with an unquiet conscience, they might then have openly with an honest fame, and beget children whom they may love truly as legitimate, and bring them godly up ...[16]

His desire to see de facto relationships regularized is deeply compassionate, demonstrating a sympathy for the plight of individuals unable to live up to the demands of celibacy, or to enjoy legitimate family life.

The extent to which Erasmus can accept the role of innovator in Europe's revolutionary thinking about Christian marriage – thinking that was to enable ministry and marriage to coexist in the Reformation – cannot be determined. But it is clear that twenty years before the "official" Reformation began, before Luther advocated clerical marriage and a new status for wedlock, Erasmus was proposing some of the crucial ideas that would allow later writers to formulate their innovative theology. In particular, his views that sexuality was of the natural order and of the essence of human nature; that marriage and the human condition were made for each other; and that celibacy was a token of the divine, rather than human, way of life and therefore appropriate only for the very few, foreshadow much of the later marriage–celibacy debate.

On the other hand, his warm evocation of the joys of married life and of parenthood, his defense of women, his elevation of companionate marriage, and his refusal to see marriage as in any sense a remedy for sin or concession to weakness, had few reverberations in contemporary thought for a century or more.

In fact, two decades later a strongly conservative approach to marriage was published – ironically, by Henry VIII. His *Assertio Septem Sacramentorum*, a defence of the seven sacraments, was written as a refutation of the Protestant writings of Martin Luther. It was for this highly orthodox document that the pope rewarded Henry with the title "Defender of the Faith."

For Henry, it was only sacramental grace, available through the sacrament of matrimony, that redeemed the sinfulness of human sexuality. This infusion of grace – described in terms of a dynamic substance – purged and sanctified the sexual act "which of its own nature defiles to punishment." It was the God-given remedy for "concupiscence," transforming human sexuality which, without it, was always base, sinful, and disgusting.[17]

Further evidence of the conflict of varying Christian views on marriage held at this time of theological turmoil is found in the writings of Martin Luther, the "father" of the Protestant Reformation. In 1523, as a wedding gift for a friend, Luther wrote his *Commentary on 1 Corinthians VII*. This famous chapter from Paul's first letter to the Corinthians had traditionally been the central biblical proof text for the priority of celibacy and the inferiority of marriage. Luther and his contemporaries would turn the tables in a dramatic way, by making this very same chapter the cornerstone for their arguments *against* celibacy, and particularly against compulsory celibacy of the clergy.[18]

In many ways, this commentary is in direct contrast to Erasmus' joyous praise of marriage. Though written as a wedding gift, marriage here is not portrayed as a happy or satisfying way of life. Rather, its description of almost every aspect of married life is in tune with the Church's long tradition of suspicion and distaste. From the beginning of his commentary, Luther makes it clear that he sees marriage as a difficult and unpleasant way of life. That, for Luther, is what St Paul meant when he began chapter seven with the words, "It is good for a man not to touch a woman." Throwing aside the traditional interpretation that this is clear proof that chastity is spiritually meritorious, Luther

47

claims that Paul refers to the earthly pleasantness of living single, for "whoever lives unmarried and celibate is relieved of all the labour and disgust which are part of the married state."[19]

Openly employing the ancient dualistic notion of human nature that had informed much of the Church's theological understanding of marriage and sexuality, Luther states that, "according to the spirit," the Christian has no need of marriage. But the Christian's flesh is "the common flesh, corrupted in Adam and Eve, filled with evil desires." Because of this "disease," marriage is a necessity even for the Christian, whose flesh "rages, burns and fructifies like that of any other man, unless he helps and controls it with the proper medicine, which is marriage."[20]

Luther suggests that even in the explicit act of procreation a married couple commits sin, a sin that is nevertheless forgiven by God because God has given permission for the married state. In earlier writings on marriage, Luther had described all sexual desire, even within marriage, as corrupting, and claimed that sexual intercourse, since the Fall, could never be without sin. Luther's understanding of married sexuality was therefore entirely conventional, and totally unreformed.[21]

But it parted company from tradition at two crucial points, and thus unwittingly offered the way forward for the ultimate reversal of Christian doctrine. Luther refuted the received view that celibacy was possible for all people, and argued that marriage was in fact physically necessary for most men, because of their fallen physical natures. The argument for clerical marriage arises, for Luther, quite naturally out of the combination of these two innovative ideas as he understands them – that celibacy is only for the very few people specially gifted by God to live chaste, and that therefore the only way for the vast majority of the clergy to control their physical natures was with the "medicine" of marriage.

The key to this argument, for Luther and those who followed him, was verse nine of chapter seven: "It is better to marry than to burn." Luther maintained that sexual passion in those lacking the God-given gift of celibacy was simply unavoidable, and could only be handled through marriage. Luther's true celibate — and they are so rare that there should be a "hundred thousand" married people for every one chaste person — felt only transitory temptation, and not the "burning" for which St Paul prescribed marriage. He condemned those who, in promoting celibacy, argued that the endurance of intense sexual frustration pleased God because of the bitterness and hardship of the suffering involved. To the contrary, this suffering was sinful, he declared, because it can be avoided through marriage.[22]

Priests, he continued, were no different from other men. To forbid them marriage was "to say that a man is not a man but is to cease being God's creature." The priestly role was not relevant to marital status. To say that a priest might not marry was to deny the holiness of marriage, Luther wrote, for marriage cannot be called "a godly thing and a holy sacrament" if it is not permitted to stand beside the holiness of the priest, otherwise "God must oppose himself."[23]

The former monk had no time for the supposed chastity of the religious orders. Better for monks to tend pigs as married men than to "torture themselves with the regulations of men and murmur and howl in the choir." In fact, married life was a more religious way of life than the cloisters, where all the necessities of life were provided. Married men must themselves provide for their wives and children, and so are compelled to trust in God.[24]

Luther expressed sympathy for those clergy living in de facto relationships, burdened with heavy consciences and the disgrace of their "wives" and children. They should be able to live honestly together, caring nothing for the pope or canon law. Describing the papal laws against clerical marriage as "the bidding of the devil," he claimed that the whole canon law would in fact "go to pieces" under the sort of church government and administration that could allow freedom of choice to the clergy. Luther seemed to be under no illusion that the law of chastity had anything but a corrupt, even financial, origin, as it ensured the full control of church property and income by church officials rather than clerical families.[25]

For a brief moment, Luther seemed to understand that the clergy wife might have more uses than merely keeping her husband from sexual sin. She could care for the "necessities of the household," he wrote. Ten years later, after five years of orderly life with his efficient and industrious wife Katherine von Bora, a former nun, he was suggesting that a married man's endless worry about money – a real obstacle to his service of God – could be lifted from the pastor by the wife. She could do the worrying herself, leaving him simply to serve God. The actual experience of clerical marriage was beginning, in a small way, to demonstrate the unreality of many of the arguments that had been used against it.[26]

Over all, though, companionship and mutual support are not important reasons for any marriage, let alone clerical marriage, in Luther's writings. Even though he pays it lip service, procreation is not the major reason. Quite simply, fallen and therefore diseased human nature needs the "medicine" of marriage to avoid sin. This nature is common to all men, including priests, and therefore priests require the remedy of marriage as much as any other men. True chastity can only be achieved with the rare gift of God, something that cannot be vowed, and even that chastity does not win a man merit in the eyes of God. It merely ensures him an earthly life free of the difficulties and disgust of married life. Yet that married life, for all its problems and inherent unavoidable sinfulness, is "of God, and pleases him well."[27]

The unchaste living of the supposedly celibate clergy and monks around him provided Luther and his fellow reformers with all the proof they needed of the truth of this case. At a time when ordination was the basic qualification for men who wanted to work in all areas of academe, government or civil service – and therefore was not necessarily linked to a life of service of God – it was highly unlikely that all clergy would feel a vocation to chastity. While historians have questioned the more extreme claims of the reformers about the level of unchastity among sixteenth-century clergy, it cannot be doubted that there was some truth in the claims. After all, in modern times, careful observers of the clergy of the Church of Rome would recognize a higher level of clerical "concubinage" around the world than would be officially acknowledged.

It is interesting, although not at all surprising, to note that for all his powerful arguments in favor of clerical marriage, Luther nevertheless found the idea psychologically disturbing, at least in the years before his own marriage. In a sermon preached at Wittenberg in 1522, he commented that the conscience needed continual "fortification" in order to cope with it. In fact, he had originally found it hard to accept that monks who had voluntarily vowed celibacy (in contrast to priests, who had no choice but to embrace it in taking on their order) could be allowed to marry. In 1521, he had exclaimed against it, declaring that "they will not push a wife on me!" By 1525, the former monk had in fact married, though there is a story (perhaps apocryphal) that he wept uncontrollably at the loss of his virginity as he consummated his marriage union.[28] Luther was a man, a priest, of his time. Centuries of teaching could not easily be swept aside.

Though for modern eyes Luther's views are still far too wedded to the ancient tradition, to his contemporaries he was outrageously radical. As has been pointed out, "here was embodied one of the most profound changes in Western civilisation in regard to the relationship between men and women."[29] Public outcry was only to be expected, as occurs when any theologians challenge current received opinion. Henry VIII – later to be much-married – hurled abuse at Luther and called his chastity into question before his marriage took place:

> ... This holy priest (whereby you may conjecture how chaste he himself is) makes it the greatest error, and greatest blindness imaginable, that priests should undertake to lead a single life. And when Christ praises those who have made themselves eunuchs for the kingdom ...[30]

After Luther's marriage, Henry's disgust knew no bounds. His marriage was no less than "lechery," which compromised all his doctrines, especially where they contradicted the Fathers. For the Fathers "were good men and of holy living, serving God in fasting, prayer and chastity." But the reformers clearly were not good men, for people could see that

> ... all of your doing began of envy and presumption, proceedeth with rancour and malice, blowen forth with pride and vainglory, and endeth in lechery. [31]

Henry's invective against Luther offers a fascinating insight into the reaction to the marriage of the clergy at this early period of the Reformation. Henry says that not only has Luther "violated" a nun, but, what is much worse, he has openly married her. This demonstrates an abominable contempt of the sacrament of matrimony, as well as of their vows of chastity. Even worse, instead of being sorry for this "heinous" deed, he openly exhorts other clergy to the same sin. [32]

As Richard Marius, one of Luther's modern biographers, has pointed out, Luther's marriage to the former nun "seemed to incarnate all the obscene jokes that had been circulating about the lecheries of religious orders for centuries," and no one was more willing to make capital out of that joke than the English polemicist Thomas More. He ridiculed these marriages of clergy and former religious, likening them to demonic orgies:

> Priests, monks, virgins, dedicated to God, now by the favour of the devil, in the church of the wicked, under the title of lawful spouses, with great pomp of demons celebrate nefarious nuptials ... [33]

But despite strong efforts of the king and his government to stop the flow of the ideas of Luther and his followers into England, those ideas nevertheless crossed the English Channel unabated. Reformed ideas were becoming widely disseminated, and Thomas More wrote again in attack. In particular, he condemned Luther for his "lechery," in increasingly sensational and salacious terms. The marriages of monks and nuns were, for More, the worst of all the reformers' heresies, robbing the reformers of any credibility they might otherwise have. If they wanted their theology taken seriously, then the reformers must recant their defense of clerical marriage.

For the modern reader, More's reaction to clerical marriage, and to Luther's in particular, seems to be at best extreme, at worst hysterical, perhaps even obsessional. In the sixteenth century, however, he was employing an invaluable polemical method. Building on the familiar ribald jokes directed against unchaste religious, More was exploiting a devastatingly simple method of ridiculing the credibility of all reformed ideas. Later the major English language defense of celibacy would employ exactly the same tactic. But behind the coarse language that drove his point home, More and other defenders of the status quo saw serious doctrinal and canonical objections to clerical marriage. Apart from any other consideration, under canon law the marriage of monk and nun, as brother and sister in Christ, was akin to incest.[34]

The historian Gordon Rupp has suggested that, for More in particular, Luther was not merely "playing foul but wrecking the very rules of the game." Rupp recalls Erasmus' comment that More had "decided to be a chaste husband rather than a licentious priest," and suggests that for a man who had had to make an agonizing choice between family life and the priesthood, this changing of the rules was intolerable.[35] Doubtless there were others like More for whom the change was also personally painful. Similarly, in recent times many intelligent older women have reacted strongly against the ordination of women in their churches. Their own lifelong acceptance of a traditional limited female role in church and society has been seriously questioned by this radical change, though most would not have identified the true source of their profound discomfort.

That the defenders of theological orthodoxy found clerical marriage such a useful and sensational weapon against the reformers – to be employed not only in attacking them personally but also in exposing their credentials as theologians — gives some indication of the cost involved for the reformers in undertaking marriage. As men of their time, they must have realized that such a reaction was inevitable. Many of the first Protestants doubtless were glad of the new dispensation that allowed them to marry for love or sexual gratification.

But others, like Luther himself, married deliberately to demonstrate their faith in this particular teaching, and for no other reason.[36] There is an irony there, surely. For although Luther came to enjoy and appreciate married life, he claimed not to have been specially troubled by sexual temptation in the monastery. By the standards of his own teaching, it seems he was constitutionally one of those very few for whom chastity was a manageable, even comfortable, way of life. He apparently did not need the "medicine" of marriage at all. But his correspondence reveals that he believed himself increasingly under pressure to do more than merely advocate marriage for other clergy and former monks. He had to embrace it himself in order to demonstrate its centrality to the Reformation doctrines.

Perhaps nothing demonstrates so graphically the truly radical nature of the reformers' doctrines of both marriage and ministry than this particular clash: while Protestants accepted marriage as the ultimate proof of their commitment to their understanding of the Gospel, their detractors could see those marriages only as the inevitable denial of it, nothing more than an obscene joke. We will turn later to an appraisal of why the marriage of the clergy was in fact so central to the reformers' theology. But first, we will look at the effect of the turning of the tables.

4

TURNING
THE TABLES

"It is now a thing worthy to be noted, that married folks are not despised of God." So the Italian reformer Peter Martyr Vermigli began his Oxford lectures, in about 1548, on the famous seventh chapter of the first letter to the Corinthians. It was a succinct and telling summary of the theological revolution that was under way, of which Martyr was a living testimony. Martyr, a priest, was also a married man, invited to England by the Archbishop of Canterbury, Thomas Cranmer. In about April 1548, a few months after his arrival, he brought his wife to join him – nearly a year before clerical marriage was first made legal in England in February 1549.

But if Martyr, and the other married reformers brought to England by Cranmer at the same time, believed firmly in the proposition that married folks are not despised of God, the good folk of Oxford thought otherwise. The townspeople were apparently in uproar over the introduction of openly married foreign reformers into their midst. Martyr and his wife had to move into secluded rooms because in their original lodgings, opening onto the street, they were subjected to "opprobrious language." Moreover the lodgings themselves had their windows broken.[1] So the disgust of married clergy already expressed by kings and courtiers continued unabated at every level of English society. For unlike the situation on the Continent, where clerical marriage was accepted relatively easily by mid-century, in England it continued to be the subject of controversy until the beginning of the seventeenth century. It took until 1604 for clerical marriage to be finally legalized in England, for the 1549 legislation had been overturned, after just a few short years, in the reign of Mary I.

But while scholars have generally assumed that these married reformers were an exceptional novelty in England – unlike on the Continent, where clergy had been openly marrying since 1522 – the evidence is that some English clergy were themselves quietly marrying by the time the high-profile foreigners arrived. After the formation of the national Church of England in 1533, following Henry VIII's formal break with Rome, pressure was clearly mounting within England for the abolition of the celibacy law. Reformed views on this and other subjects had powerfully infiltrated the English thought-world. The campaign against the monasteries, which culminated in the 1539 *Act for the Dissolution of the Greater Monasteries*, had been strongly orchestrated as an attack on the moral dangers of enforced celibacy. The royal visitations of the monasteries in 1535 and 1536 had been at least partly designed to gather evidence that would bring celibacy into disrepute. Only four of the more than 120 religious houses in the north of England examined by Richard Layton and Thomas Legh, for example, provided any record of a crime or misdemeanor committed by the monastics that was not sexual in nature.[2]

The first major English assault on priestly, rather than monastic, celibacy had come at the same time, in 1534, from the pen of Robert Barnes. Barnes (1495–1540), today regarded as a minor figure of the English Reformation, was a significant reformer in the eyes of his generation. A former Augustinian friar who never married, he wrote a chapter advocating clerical marriage to add to a general work he had published three years earlier. Perhaps in the new climate of reform in England, now newly separated from Rome, he believed clerical marriage was a real possibility, as it had not been in 1531. His essay is a careful, biblically based argument that was later recognized as being the theological pioneer of much of the later writing in defense of clerical marriage.[3]

It is interesting that Barnes goes to great lengths in this chapter to assure his readers that he himself is not married, hotly denying rumors that he has a wife. If he had, he would not have dared to tackle the subject, he asserts, for it would rob his writing of credibility.[4] But the fact that Barnes had to deny that he was married suggests that, by 1534, clerical marriage was already a reality in England. Indeed, Barnes offers some direct evidence that this was the case when he complains about England's persecution of married priests. It is an extraordinary piece of evidence that has been totally overlooked by historians, making it worth repeating in full:

> Where is there one man in England, that hath so great love, and reverence to the holy state of matrimony, that he should keep a married priest in his house? But priests that live unlawfully against God's law, and man's law, and against all honesty, and moral virtue, be in every man's houses and company ... Alas for pity, what shall I say to the affections of men's hearts, that thus can wink (I will not say allow) at such abominable things. Yea, and the self-same men shall be most extreme, and cruel unto a poor simple priest, that of a good heart towards God's ordinance, marrieth a lawful wife. This priest, I say, shall neither have meat, nor drink of them, nor yet no office of charity. But the other sort shall be exalted, and set up in all honour and kept in reverence and estimation. And why? Because as they say they be good and clean fellows, and loveth a piece of flesh well. These blasphemous words have I heard diverse times and many ...[5]

This evidence reveals that in 1534 not only was there a growing number of married clergy in England but the persecution they encountered was social rather than legal or ecclesiastical. It is clear too that Barnes regarded these unions to be completely lawful, though technically they were still subject to the invalidity conferred by the 1139 decree of the Second Lateran Council.

Presumably the clergy who married utilized some form of marriage rite. At a time when the systematic recording of marriages was confined to local parish registers – and was therefore at the discretion of sympathetic colleagues – this was far easier than we might imagine.

The defence of clerical marriage, even at this early stage, was more than an academic exercise, even for an unmarried writer. It was a defense of the clergy who were marrying, and suffering for it. This was to be the pattern over the ensuing decades, as persecution in varying degrees caused a succession of English reformers to write and publish in defense of clerical marriage. In doing so, they left future theologians the tools to piece together both the overt and the underlying reasons for this extraordinary shift in the understanding of human sexuality.

It is tempting to take literally Barnes' mention of "poor, simple priests" and to assume that it was only humble, uneducated curates and the like who married before clerical marriage was first legalized in 1549. However, the case of one of the first Protestant martyrs of the reign of Mary I suggests otherwise. Dr Rowland Taylor, Rector of Hadley, Suffolk, was not merely a country parson. A doctor of civil and canon law, he has been described as a "man of learning, a great preacher," who had left the household of Thomas Cranmer to take up his parish, which he transformed into a thoroughly Protestant center. The martyrologist John Foxe records that, during the examination of Dr Taylor for heresy in 1555, the fact of his marriage was one of the first "heresies" leveled against him. Taylor's reply, that he was indeed married and had had nine children "all in lawful matrimony," indicates that he must have married at least by the early 1540s, if not considerably earlier.[6]

Still more telling was the marriage of Thomas Cranmer, which is supposed to have taken place in Nuremberg in 1532. Even though he did not expect to be made Archbishop of Canterbury that very year, he was no lowly curate! Archdeacon, king's chaplain and ambassador when he traveled to Nuremberg on the king's business, he expected a reasonably swift return to

England, and presumably expected it would be acceptable to return with a wife. If he did marry then – and it is by no means certain that he did – it would be indicative both of the climate of opinion in England at the time, and of the expectation that the celibacy law would soon be relaxed there.[7]

If the climate was favorable early in the 1530s, it was soon to change. In 1539, in a reactionary mood, Henry VIII turned his back on the gentle reformation simmering in his new national church. In the ferocious *Six Articles Act*, he demanded a return to the old status quo, insisting on a belief in transubstantiation, communion in one kind, private masses, auricular confession, chastity vows, and clerical celibacy – the main targets of Reformation zeal. It is significant that two of the six "articles" deal with clerical marriage and vows of chastity, indicating the importance to the Protestant cause of marriage for priests and former monastics. Under the terms of the Act, the sentence for any clergyman twice convicted of marriage was death – more severe than any conviction for either fornication or adultery. A year later the Act was amended, removing the death penalty for marriage; but that such extreme measures were even contemplated indicates that clergy must have been marrying in significant numbers in England by this stage.[8]

Protestant-minded bishops such as Cranmer and Latimer initially opposed the provisions of the Act in Parliament, but were eventually left with no choice but to vote with the king. Two bishops, one of whom was Latimer, later resigned their bishoprics over it.[9] But the majority of the English bishops supported it, a fact that would inflame the anger of reforming clergy. In this time of reaction, numbers of these English Protestants felt compelled to flee into exile on the Continent. Those who remained in England, still preaching the virtues of clerical marriage among other "heresies," were forced to recant.[10] The Protestant Reformation in England had met full-scale resistance; the future for the reformers was bleak.

Not unexpectedly, the Act was the cause of the publication of a wave of writings, both home-grown and foreign, defending

Reformation principles, and not least clerical marriage. They included an English translation of the work of an influential Continental reformer, Philipp Melanchthon (1497–1560). *A Very Godly Defence ... Defending the Marriage of Priests*, originally written in Latin and directed to the King of England, was translated by the exiled George Joye (1495?–1553), who later went on to write his own "defence". This work specifically targeted Bishop Stephen Gardiner of Winchester, who most of the English reformers believed was responsible for the *Six Articles Act*.[11]

The Melanchthon book contains some fascinating commentary on the *Six Articles Act* and its motivation. It was, he said, "bloody tyranny" for both man and wife to be hanged for marriage, for "godly poor men and their wives" to be hanged "like thieves and murderers," and a cruelty unworthy of the Church to "hang, burn and slay men for marrying their lawful wives." The reasons for this monstrous attack on clerical marriage are not religious, he claims, but secular, for unmarried clergy are far more useful in the households of kings, nobles and even bishops than men encumbered by wives and families. He warns that by maintaining "wiveless chastity," princes and bishops are inadvertently upholding the power of the pope. Enforced chastity is, he says, the "strong sinew to hold fast and keep still all the rest of the whole impiety and mischief of the Bishop of Rome."[12]

Overall, Melanchthon's work is a calm, cogent and well-argued dissertation that tackles carefully and specifically some of the key issues in the academic debate, as we will see later. Melanchthon lived far away, and was not immediately involved. Joye, however, possibly in exile himself because of marriage, penned his own tract in considerable anger and bitterness, recording the suffering of clergy families "drawn in sunder [sic] as it were with wild horses," unable even to remain resident in the same town.[13] The language is strong and polemical, as he accuses the bishops of supporting the *Six Articles Act* so that clergy can continue to enjoy the pleasures of sexual license without the responsibility or expense of marriage. Like many of the reformers, he was angered by the hypocrisy that winked at any amount of immoral clerical sexual activity, but which inspired persecution of married clergy.[14]

Later in the reign of Henry VIII, John Bale, another priest forced into exile because of marriage, lashed out at what he saw as the farce of enforced celibacy. Bale (1495–1563), later to be Bishop of Ossory in Ireland, had married shortly after his conversion to Protestantism and the renunciation of his vows as a Carmelite monk in 1529. With his "poor wife and children," he fled to Germany in 1540, where he wrote a catalog of lurid tales about the "unchaste practices" of "English votaries." Written in a coarse, sensationalist style, his book comes close to being sixteenth-century pornography, dwelling in detail on endless stories of gross immorality among clergy and monastics over the centuries. His aim is clearly to demolish the notion that celibacy is a way of life holier than that of marriage.[15]

This insistence that celibacy was the holy way of life for the clergy may have been the public reason offered for persecuting married clergy, but there are indications that it was not the only reason. While recognizing that Joye is clearly biased and therefore not necessarily an accurate reporter, we can see he nevertheless offers an interesting reason for the Parliament's defense of clerical celibacy. The Duke of Norfolk – who introduced the *Six Articles Act* into Parliament – was, Joye claims, principally concerned that clergy, if allowed to marry, might choose the daughters of noblemen or gentlemen, thus securing their dowries and their lands. "At last ye shall see the bishops have all our lands," Joye quotes him as saying.[16] There is in fact corroborating evidence that this lay behind Henry VIII's opposition to clerical marriage. A correspondent to a foreign court at about the same time claimed that, of all the Protestant tenets, the king most disliked clergy marriage, because "the priests would tyrannise over princes themselves, and make benefices hereditary."[17]

Both the king and the Duke of Norfolk, if we can believe these reports, were operating out of the very reasons historians have identified as underlying the imposition of clerical celibacy in the Gregorian period, which we have already discussed. Married clergy inevitably acted out of a set of loyalties different to those of celibates, because of their responsibility to their wives, children, and wider kinship networks. They had concerns about money and property, and were not automatically available to serve pope, king or nobleman. In Norfolk's imagination, they posed a real threat to the stability of the aristocracy, first by infiltrating the carefully guarded network of great families, and in time by creating a new, rival network.

For whatever reason, the die was cast for the rest of Henry VIII's reign. A married clergy was out of the question, and we can only imagine the extent of the anger and anguish felt by clergy forcibly separated from their families under pain of severe punishment, or compelled to flee into exile. Clergy marriage had become a highly charged emotional issue, which gave a sharp edge to any academic discussion both then and in the future.

In this dangerous environment, what became of the most senior churchman in the land, the Archbishop of Canterbury? As other clergy were forcibly separated from their families, or fled into exile, Thomas Cranmer continued in his role untouched. He had supposedly married during a visit to Nuremberg in 1532, but the only extant reference to his marriage that predates his inquisition before his execution dates the marriage around June 1550. John Stumphius, a young Swiss student studying in England, reported by letter to Heinrich Bullinger that "there is also the greatest hope as to religion, for the archbishop of Canterbury has lately married a wife." Accepting the earlier date for his marriage given at Cranmer's trial, historians have generally assumed that the comment refers to the point at which he made his wife's existence public.

But this poses more problems than it solves. Why should Cranmer wait until June 1550 to reveal the fact of his marriage, when clerical marriage had been legalized in February 1549? And when foreign reformers such as Peter Martyr and Francisco Dryander had openly brought their wives to England even before that date? Martin Bucer and Paul Fagius, two of the visitors, reported to the ministers of Strasbourg a happy social gathering at Lambeth Palace in April 1549 with the other reformers – a gathering that included their wives. Though she was supposed to be German and a connection of the reformer Andreas Osiander, there is no mention of Mrs Cranmer at all. Where was she?

Certainly her whereabouts a decade previously during the enforcement of the *Six Articles Act* taxed Cranmer's earliest biographers. Their accounts differ markedly in their attempts to explain where she was, and why the Archbishop escaped the full force of the new law. The record of Cranmer's life compiled by his secretary, Ralph Morice, does not mention her, but Foxe, who drew on this account, claims that she stayed in England throughout that period "by secret consent of the King's Majesty thereunto." The Elizabethan Archbishop of Canterbury, Matthew Parker, gave a different version of events. He said that Cranmer had sent her back to Germany and that the king, in discovering Cranmer's secret, had treated him leniently. Neither account, however, explains why her presence should not have been made public at least by February 1549. Cranmer's marriage remains a mystery; whatever the truth might be, it did nothing to advance or help the cause of clerical marriage at this critical period.[18]

The death of Henry VIII in 1547 and the accession of his sickly young son Edward VI with his Protestant backers gave the Reformation a new beginning in England. Within a few short years, the independent English Church had its first Prayer Book, as well as many other innovations that would later provide the groundwork for the solid gains of the Elizabethan Settlement.

Both Convocation (the meeting of the clergy) and the House of Commons approved priestly marriage speedily in 1547. Convocation agreed by three to one that all laws and canons against clerical marriage should be revoked. But the House of Lords was not so easily persuaded. The opposition came principally from the bishops – many of whom presumably had supported the *Six Articles Act* – but legislation permitting marriage for priests both before and after ordination finally became law on 19 February 1549. The preamble to the legislation offers an accurate summary of the attitudes toward clerical marriage that prevailed throughout the lengthy debate on the subject, and is worth quoting:

> Although it were not only better for the estimation of priests, and other ministers in the Church of God, to live chaste, sole, and separate from the company of women and the bond of marriage, but also thereby they might the better intend to the administration of the gospel, and be less intricated and troubled with the charge of a household, being free and unburdened from the care and cost of finding wife and children, and that it were most to be wished that they would willingly and of their selves endeavour themselves to a perpetual chastity and abstinence from the use of women: Yet forasmuch as the contrary hath rather been seen, and such uncleanness of living, and other great inconveniences, not meet to be rehearsed, have followed of compelled chastity, and of such laws as have prohibited those (such persons) the godly use of marriage; it were better and rather to be suffered in the commonwealth, that those which could not contain, should, after the counsel of Scripture, live in holy marriage, than feignedly abuse with worse enormity outward chastity or single life ... [19]

At least in the public rhetoric, then, the marriage of priests was no more than a grudging concession to pragmatic concerns. Marriage, for all that it was described as both "holy" and "godly," was nevertheless still a regrettable way of life for clergy and, in effect, something less than holy. Celibacy clearly retained its ancient preeminence, its aura of true holiness. The corresponding denigration of women echoes strongly through this preamble, for the "use of women" (sexual intercourse) and indeed the "company of women" are preferably to be avoided if at all possible. Throughout the tracts defending clerical marriage, sexual intercourse is almost always called "the use of women" – a telling euphemism indeed.

Here is no glowing affirmation of the goodness of marriage and of human sexuality, but rather an admission that marriage was the only way to control wayward human urges. Permission for clerical marriage constitutes a revolutionary reordering of the Church's rules based on its exaltation of chastity, but does not yet introduce a fundamental overturning of that exaltation. The prime motivation, according to the preamble, is the public scandal of the lives of the clergy, which can be overcome only by the control of marriage. The reason for the change is not primarily a theological reassessment of sex and marriage, but rather a concern for the godly living of the clergy. As we will see, that was the result of theological reassessment of a different order.

The actual passing of the legislation did not of itself open the floodgates to clerical marriage. As we have seen, the clergy were already marrying in significant numbers. Matthew Parker, later to be Archbishop of Canterbury, was Master of Corpus Christi College, Cambridge, when he married Margaret Harlston in June 1547, according to his own memorandum. However, in recording her death in 1570, he notes that she had lived with him "some twenty-six years," which suggests a marriage date closer to 1544. Quite possibly he had married her secretly during the reign of Henry, and made the marriage public some months after Henry's death, when it was clear that the succession was in Protestant hands. Many more clergy may well have made existing marriages public in the same way, none of them waiting for formal legislation to be passed. Married exiles returned from abroad as soon as Henry was dead, bringing their wives and families with them. Miles Coverdale, the Bible translator, soon to be appointed Bishop of Exeter, hurried home with his wife Elizabeth; John Bale returned with his family, to be appointed to the living of Bishopstoke, Hampshire.[20]

So why did Peter Martyr find himself subject to such public abuse in Oxford in 1548? Perhaps he was singled out because he defended clerical marriage and other Reformation doctrines in his first lectures at the university. His student Simler records that the masters of the Oxford Colleges at first simply kept their students from attending his lectures. But once he had "condemned their vows of sole life, and that consequently upon occasion of the Apostles words ... they thought it was not for them to be any longer quiet." Another factor was the agitation of his predecessor as Regius Professor, Dr Richard Smith, who had been deposed by the new king. Martyr recorded that Smith was often present at his lectures, taking notes. Smith, who was later to write a defense of celibacy against Martyr, took particular exception to the fact of Martyr's marriage. Much to the Italian's distress, he described Martyr's wife as his "harlot."[21]

There can be little doubt that Martyr's controversial lectures at Oxford were the beginning of efforts in the new reign to have clerical marriage, though not yet legalized, accepted theologically. From that telling opening sentence – "it is now a thing worthy to be noted, that married folks are not despised of God" – it seems Martyr, newly arrived from the Continent, believed that Protestant theology had already by that stage produced a considerable shift in thought on the nature of marriage. The response he received, however, must have made it clear that no such thing had yet happened in England, for all that there were now numerous married clergy. The preamble to the legislation must have underlined the limited nature of the English understanding at that time.

Given the treatment meted out to Peter Martyr, it is no wonder that Cranmer was anxious to provide more ammunition for the propaganda war even after the legislation had been passed. In 1549 his chaplain, John Ponet, published a work defending the marriage of priests "by Scripture and ancient writers." In this small-scale, tightly written tract, Ponet stresses that he is writing not only to inform both laity and clergy about clerical marriage, but also to "quiet the consciences of many, which be not yet fully instructed and resolved, in this point." This suggests a high level of controversy over the issue, which is hardly surprising.

In particular, Ponet deals with an aspect of the contemporary debate that was obviously pressing. Had English priests taken a vow of celibacy at the time of their priestly ordination? It was an area of much dispute, as the upholders of clerical celibacy claimed that all priests ordained under the old dispensation had vowed celibacy and that marriage, accordingly, was not an option for them. Clearly there was no unequivocal celibacy vow in the ordinal used in pre-Reformation England, as the argument centered on whether taking general priestly vows implied a commitment to celibacy. Reform-minded clergy, naturally, insisted that there was no such commitment on the part of English priests, and that they, therefore, were free to marry in consequence of the change in the law.[22]

Such concerns were soon to be overtaken, however. Edward VI's brief reign came to an abrupt end in 1553, when he was succeeded by his half-sister, Mary I. A devout Catholic, Mary implemented a fierce reversal of the Protestant Reformation, resulting in the deaths of nearly 300 Protestants, including Archbishop Cranmer. Among the catalog of changes she introduced was the outlawing once more of all clerical marriage.

By the time Mary repealed the 1549 legislation, as many as a quarter of the clergy in some parts of England had married. Few of them, it seems, escaped the provisions that followed this repeal. Secular clergy were required to separate from their wives, and to leave their parishes. Those who had once belonged to religious orders (and of whose solemn vows of chastity there could therefore be no doubt) were treated more severely, being forced to divorce their wives and undergo humiliating public rituals of penance. It has been estimated that as many as one-sixth of the benefices of England were affected by these wholesale deprivations of clergy. The only clergy couples who survived were those who fled abroad, like John Ponet and his wife, or went into hiding, like Matthew Parker and his.[23]

The level of dislocation and distress suffered by so many people, particularly the abandoned wives and children, can only be guessed at. For some who had married in Henry's reign, it was a second period of humiliation. The bitterness and anger many felt at such treatment, specially those who had married openly, in good faith, and with the blessing of both Convocation and the law of England, resounded through the next wave of tracts written to defend clerical marriage.

Matthew Parker, whose *Defence* was substantially written during the Marian years (though it was not published until 1567), recorded his dismay at the way lawful marriages were treated. The process of dismissal was careless, cavalier and often unlawful, he claimed. Many clergy, including himself, were tricked out of rightful income, while those prepared to recant and move on to new parish livings were properly paid. Many wives were left destitute, for though they were supposedly divorced, few men believed they were truly free to marry again.[24]

Parker's *Defence* was not merely a record of these unhappy events. It was written primarily in response to a publication designed to defend the deprivation and punishment of the married clergy. Thomas Martin, a civil lawyer, published his work, quite possibly with official sanction, in 1554, shortly after the deprivations began. The only substantial, full-scale defence of celibacy written during the English Reformation, its full title is an accurate guide to its contents and polemical purpose: *A Traictise Declaring and Plainly Proving, that the Pretensed Marriage of Priests, and Professed Persons, is no Marriage, but Altogether Unlawful, and in All Ages, and All Countries of Christendom, Both Forbidden and Also Punished*. The deprivations were justified, then, on the grounds that clerical marriage was a contradiction in terms, and no more than a pretense.

Mary's reign was short, however, and the Catholic "reaction" she instituted came to an abrupt end itself with the accession of her half-sister, Elizabeth I, in 1558. But if the married clergy were hopeful of a speedy reversal of their fortunes, they were much mistaken. Elizabeth's limited Protestantism did not extend to a sanguine view of clerical marriage – far from it. She disliked the very idea heartily, and consistently refused to restore parliamentary legislation to put its legality beyond question. The result was that Mary's prohibitive legislation remained on the statute books of England until the reign of James I, when in 1604 a new law finally gave the marriage of priests lasting and unequivocal legal sanction in England.

Clergy were, however, given grudging permission to marry by Elizabeth's Injunctions of 1559. But it was a patronizing, limited permission. They could only marry with the permission of the bishop and two justices of the peace, who were required to make "good examination" of the proposed union. Bishops needed permission from both their archbishop and commissioners appointed by the queen. Even so, the bride had to have the permission of her parents or "her master or mistress, where she serveth ..." These precautions were intended, according to the Injunctions, to prevent the "offence" and "slander" being caused the Church by the "lack of discreet and sober behaviour in many ministers," both in choosing their wives and living with them.

The Injunctions seemed to assume that only women from the servant class would marry priests. But the fact that permission was also required from parents for women who were beyond the age of legal majority may have been included to quiet fears that clergy might marry the daughters of the gentry, as expressed by members of the nobility at the time of the *Six Articles Act*.[25]

The Injunctions provided at best only limited permission, and were dependent on the sovereign's personal will alone, as long as they were not supported by an Act of Parliament. The insecurity of such permission was demonstrated as early as August 1561, when the queen banned clerical wives from residing in cathedral precincts and university colleges, causing real consternation among married priests. Bishop Cox of Ely, whose wife had been among the first clergy wives resident at Oxford, complained to Matthew Parker, now Archbishop of Canterbury, that the adversaries were rejoicing and the "godly ministers" discouraged at such a decision.

Sir William Cecil, the queen's principal secretary, warned Parker of Elizabeth's antipathy to married clergy. "Her Majesty continueth very evil affected to the state of matrimony in the clergy," he wrote to him on 12 August 1561. He added that if he, Cecil, were not "therein very stiff," the Queen would openly condemn and forbid it. The ban on wives in cathedrals and colleges had been a means of placating her, he implied.[26]

Parker himself, however, must have tackled the Queen personally on the subject, although with little success. He was deeply shocked by the interview, reporting to Cecil:

> I was in an horror to hear such words to come from her
> mild nature and Christianly learned conscience, as she
> spoke concerning God's holy ordinance and institution
> of matrimony.

While wives of horsekeepers, porters, pantlers, and butlers could "have their cradles going," the wives of the clergy, the queen's "unfeigned orators," could not. [27]

But the real fear was that there was worse to come, possibly even the outright ban Cecil had warned of. The queen, Parker reports, had regretted ever appointing married priests to high office, and had "traduced" Parker and his colleagues as

> beasts without knowledge to Godward, in using this
> liberty of his word, as men of effrenate [sic]
> intemperancy, without discretion of any godly
> disposition worthy to serve in our state.

Parker, normally mild-mannered and accommodating to his queen's religious idiosyncrasies, was uncharacteristically determined that she would not have her way in this matter. The clergy would fiercely resist any attempt to restrict clerical marriage any further, he said, not shrinking "to offer their blood to the defence of Christ's verity." His response is hardly surprising, after the agonizing vacillations of the previous reigns. Too many clergy had already endured enough on that score.[28]

So the Injunctions of 1559 were no guarantee that Elizabeth would not at some future stage change her mind. Such an ambiguous position was no commendation of clerical marriage to a society that had so recently witnessed the wholesale deprivations and public penances during the reign of Mary. Letters written to leading Continental reformers in the 1560s report the situation as yet another example of the unreformed nature of the Church of England. In a letter to Heinrich Bullinger in July 1566, Laurence Humphrey and Thomas Sampson note the lack of legislation and its consequence: some people, they write, regard the children of clergy as illegitimate.[29]

As the letters to the Continent suggest, the dubious legal situation in the first decade of Elizabeth's reign ensured continuing controversy on the subject. Three major defenses of clerical marriage were published during this troubled decade. Each of them had actually been written during the reign of Mary, when publication was impossible. New prefaces and other additions, however, record the nature of the controversy in this, its last major stage in the history of the Church of England.

John Veron, whose *A Strong Defence of the Marriage of Priests …* was published in London in 1562, was a Frenchman who had settled in England in about 1536. Whether or not he was married is not known, but he was deprived of his parish in 1554 during Mary's reign, when he was styled as a "seditious preacher." He spent the rest of her reign imprisoned in the Tower of London, which suggests he was accused of something more serious than marriage. In Elizabeth's reign, he was a frequent preacher at Paul's Cross in London, the outdoor pulpit of many leading reformers. In 1561, two men had to do public penance for accusing Veron of being "taken with a wench"![30]

The preface to Veron's book is most revealing. He identifies the opponents of clerical marriage in the new reign as no longer the "Papists," but rather those who "seem to be earnest savourers of the Scriptures." These people agree it is lawful for priests to marry by God's Word, but say it is "not expedient, that they should have wives." These Protestant opponents offer two principal objections. The married clergy will be too distracted by their wives and their "houses full of children" to "apply their learning, and give themselves to heavenly contemplation." They would thus not be able to feed their flocks with "wholesome doctrine." Second, marriage would make the clergy covetous, so that the poor would no longer be helped.

Veron counters the first argument with answers derived from Luther; wives in fact can lift domestic cares from their husbands. And besides, with the fires of sexual desire quenched by marriage, priests are more able to apply their learning, and give themselves to heavenly contemplation. As to feeding the people with the heavenly food of God's Word,

> there have been more godly sermons made in one year, by faithful married ministers, since our Sovereign Lady Queen Elizabeth did come in than were made in all Queen Mary's time, by those wifeless and virgin priests.

Veron's reply to the charge that married clergy will cause poverty is very illuminating. Do not blame clergy families, he writes, for it is those who argue against clerical marriage who are the "cause the realm is full of poverty." There is more reason to charge with covetousness those who hold office under the crown, he argues, hinting strongly that the opposition to clerical marriage comes once more from the nobility. If Veron has correctly identified them, these grounds are closely related to those discerned in 1539. They are plainly not theological, but indicate fear of a new, rival landed class.[31]

Parker was so disturbed by the threat to clerical marriage in Elizabeth's reign that he went so far as to suggest that God would directly punish those who treated with contempt God's institutions, such as marriage. God will "surely plague them all, whatsoever they be, which despise them," he writes, hinting at dire consequences for the queen herself if she banned clerical marriage outright. He had directly blamed the sour failure of Queen Mary's childless marriage, and indeed the many other catastrophes of her reign, on her "open contempt of true matrimony".[32]

Clerical marriage was not, however, totally banned during Elizabeth's reign. The ban in colleges and cathedral precincts –

which persisted until the nineteenth century – was as far as Elizabeth went in the end. In fact, clerical marriage was given a degree of security when it was allowed in Article 32 of the Church of England's Thirty-nine Articles of Religion, its continuing formal standard of faith, approved by Parliament in 1571. This must have given clerical marriage considerably more status than it had had so far under Elizabeth, and no further attempts to disallow it are recorded. Parliament's acceptance of the Articles – nine years after they had been approved by the Archbishops, bishops and clergy of England – effectively marked the end of the long and distressing controversy. The subject continued to surface in sermons and in general defenses of the reformed Church of England for the remainder of Elizabeth's reign, but the fire of debate by then had gone.[33]

The English controversy, from the 1520s to the 1570s, had not been confined to theologians, noblemen and parliamentarians. Barnes wrote of the low regard in which married clergy were generally held in society. Ponet pointed to considerable lay discomfort at the idea. Students and townspeople alike resented Peter Martyr's marital status. The impact the Marian deprivations and accompanying penances must have had on public opinion cannot be disregarded. The consequent anomalous position of married clergy in Elizabeth's reign, and the queen's own personal antipathy, could only have reinforced the opinion that clerical marriages were, at the least, distasteful.

Court records, as well as episcopal visitation articles, suggest that clergy marriages were, to many people, a reason to show disrespect to the clergy, who became a popular target for crude jokes and ribaldry. The 1571 record of Robert Long of Salcott, who claimed that "ministers' wives were whores and their children bastards," is by no means rare; it is in fact typical of many recorded comments. The Catholic polemical work, *De Origine ac Progressu Schismatis Anglicani Liber*, first published in Cologne in 1585, was, despite its obvious bias, not far from echoing popular English sentiment on the matter. Its editor, recusant priest Edward Rishton, in his addition to the original text by Nicolas Sander, comments:

> Even the Protestants, to say nothing of Catholics, would not give them [priests] their daughters in marriage; so they regarded it as something disgraceful to be, or to be said to be, the wife of a priest. Then according to the law of the land, these marriages are not yet lawful, the issue are bastards, and the wife and children obtain neither rank nor honour in the state from the rank of the father ... neither archbishop nor bishop, nor any other prelate, if married, can give any rank or precedence to his wife, who is no better than an unmarried woman.
>
> Accordingly, the Queen herself never receives these women in court, not even those who are said to be the wives of archbishops. The wives of the nobility avoid them also, and they confine themselves to the houses of those who have taken them into them. These marriages being attended by these inconveniences, hardly any honest woman could be found who would become the wife of even the highest dignitaries, who were therefore forced to marry whom they could get.[34]

To this day, the rank of peerage carried by English bishops and archbishops is not shared by their wives.

The writer adds that from the first, the married priests were careless or unlucky, for "almost all of them married women of tainted reputation." Whatever public and Catholic opinion might have been on the sort of woman who would become a priest's wife, there is however no evidence that the first generation of clerical wives were not respectable women. A study of the marital patterns of the Elizabethan bishops, of whom at least fifty-five out of seventy-six married despite the social limitations, has concluded that their wives were mostly the daughters of minor gentry, small traders, and of fellow clerics.[35] A kind of "priestly tribalism" developed in the sixteenth and seventeenth centuries with the intermarriage of clerical families. The case of the five daughters of the Elizabethan Bishop William Barlow of Chichester, all of whom married either bishops or their close relatives, is an extreme but interesting example of this "tribalism." It may well reflect social limitations forced on clergy by a still-suspicious public.[36]

The first generations of married clergy in the sixteenth century were subjected to the full onslaught of the hatred and suspicion of human sexuality bred by the long centuries of the exaltation of celibacy. It was an ugly legacy, revealed nowhere more powerfully than in the treatment of these unfortunate couples. It demonstrated explicitly that the celibacy ideal embodied the notion that holiness and sexual expression could not coexist.

Yet the reformers themselves, who were victims of such harsh treatment from many quarters for their marriages, were often ambivalent about the link between sex and holiness. What was the compelling reason that caused them to marry, and so court bodily danger and intense personal unpopularity?

5

WHY A
MARRIED PRIESTHOOD?

By the end of the sixteenth century, marriage for the clergy was well established in England. A profound theological and social revolution had taken place. Clerical marriage was still not totally respectable, however. It would take another century or so before clergy wives lost their original tainted reputation and became instead paragons of virtue, the exemplars of female respectability and piety par excellence. By then, marriage had become the normative lifestyle for Anglican clergy, as it already was for their Protestant counterparts on the Continent. Anglicanism, unlike other Protestant traditions, would nevertheless always retain a respect for clerical celibacy, perhaps as a direct consequence of the long period of debate and ambivalence.

For the first generations of married clergy, marriage was problematic, even if the violent opposition of the early years had died down. So what was the impetus that drove them to bring such dishonor on themselves? Quite possibly, the answer is simple: they wanted to get married. The powerful human drive for intimacy, companionship, and sexual fulfillment might have been quite sufficient. Today, most who argue for a married clergy in the Church of Rome would not hesitate to offer this reason. But in the sixteenth century, after long centuries of the virtually uncontested exaltation of sexual denial, it was not so straightforward.

The reformers, as men of their time, had to offer substantial theological reasons for such a profound change, to convince themselves as much as anyone else. We would expect such a change to be grounded in a major rethinking of attitudes to sexuality, to the extent that the reformers could confidently assert that marriage was of equal status to celibacy in Christian understanding. But that is not the case. With rare exceptions, the reformers continued to uphold the traditional scale of values that placed celibacy unequivocally above marriage. We must look elsewhere for their justification for this momentous change in church order.

The long and tortuous debate on clerical marriage in England in the sixteenth century – marked by the brutality of the treatment meted out to married clergy at certain points – ensured a vigorous defense on the part of the reformers. Over the best part of sixty years, as we have seen, they published "defences" of clerical marriage as propaganda for their cause. These tracts and other publications were polemical, and we would be wrong to expect them necessarily to reveal the true reasons that drove individual reformers to advocate change. In this paper war, they would have been ill-advised to use anything but the tactics most likely to persuade their opponents. Nevertheless, the tracts provide invaluable materials from which we can tease out the reformers' underlying imperatives.

The obvious place to start is with their views on sexuality, as any theology of marriage, celibacy, or even divorce or contraception, is ultimately built on this prior ground. Almost without exception, the reformers' views on sexuality alert us to the ambiguities and uncertainties inherent in their understanding of marriage. As we shall see, these views were in part formulated in order to support their justification for clerical marriage, and bear what we might call evidence of the stretch marks! To permit clergy to marry, they had to establish a level of acceptance of sexual activity; they did not decide that clergy could marry because they had first discovered that sex was good. Far from it.

Their overall attitude to human sexuality can perhaps best be summed up in the Pauline phrase, "it is better to marry than to burn." Marriage was, first and foremost, a "remedy" for sin. The reformers' most common metaphor for marital sexual activity was medicinal – that it was a cure or preventative for sinful sex. Marriage "cured" the intense sexual "burning" that would otherwise drive a man to sin and so, in a sense that surely St Paul did not mean, to burn in the fires of hell.

This telling metaphor indicates all too clearly that the reformers, almost to a man, understood the sex drive as being diseased. In common with the long tradition that had advocated chastity, the reformers saw it as a danger, a threat, to purity and holiness. This is perhaps nowhere more clearly spelt out than by Robert Barnes, when he says his doctrine is:

> use to your comfort, those creatures and remedies with
> thanksgiving, that God hath appointed, and therewith
> be you content, and reckon not yourselves wiser than
> God, in helping and curing your diseases.[1]

For Philipp Melanchthon, marriage is necessary for the "bridling" of passions otherwise uncontrollable, so that the more men struggle to control themselves without marriage, "the more nature moveth and boileth forth." That the remedy itself is God-given is proved by an appeal to St Paul, who commanded that these "perilous burnings" be "remedied and cooped with just and holy matrimony."[2] For John Veron, marriage is the "lawful water to quench the fire of concupiscence."[3] For Matthew Parker, marriage is a "port" for those molested with "storms of temptation."[4]

And yet, the reformers also claimed that the sex drive *was* God-given, and that marriage was holy! They were positively defensive about its innate goodness. For, according to both Barnes and Veron, sex was a natural force or inclination, comparable to hunger or thirst and, as such, an integral part of human nature.[5] George Joye identified God as the instigator of the sexual urge, who "by his first firm creation with his everlasting almighty word hath engraven and ingrafted it in the nature of man and woman."[6]

To Melanchthon, human nature was so created that "it must needs be fertile and fruitful," while for Barnes, the very fact that the writer of 1 Timothy 3:4 expected a bishop to be a married man with children proved that "the conjunction and copulation" between husband and wife was "godly and virtuous." In a terse marginal note he comments: "children be not gotten with looking on woman only"![7]

Again and again, the reformers quoted Hebrews 13:4: "Marriage is honourable in all, and the bed undefiled" (AV). The point that marriage was God-ordained was relatively easy for the reformers to establish. They began with the "marriage" of Adam and Eve in the Garden of Eden. Thomas Becon even depicted God as being literally the minister at this first marriage; by contrast, celibate orders were merely the work of men like St Francis, "a very simple man and a plain idiot." Jesus' first miracle was at a wedding, Becon pointed out. How the "enemies of God's truth would … have bragged of the matter" if Jesus had instead been present at the profession of a nun or the first mass of a priest, Becon said, in a breathtaking anachronism.[8]

But the sex drive implanted by God in Creation was not the sex drive that needed marriage to contain it. In common with the centuries of Christian teaching based on the theology of Augustine of Hippo, the reformers believed that the sex instinct, as originally implanted by God, had just one godly purpose, and that was procreation. Sex for any other purpose, even within marriage, was in some way diseased. And the cause of this disease was the Fall of Man. It was the Fall that had caused the natural and God-given inclination to sexual activity – which in humankind's innocency was "without fault" – to "run riot." This was the cause of the "burning," of the overwhelming temptation to sin, for which God ordained marriage as remedy.

Modern readers might be tempted to see this "burning" as encompassing all the perverted and ugly sexual sins that mar human life, all the evil that results from amoral sexual license and violence and abuse of the worst kind. Certainly the reformers, influenced by the unavoidable naïvety of their time, included these sins within the ambit of the remedy of marriage, fully believing that conjugal relations would "cure" even these ills. But they also included within the need of "cure" all that we would recognize as the legitimate and wholesome sexual expression between a married couple. Quite simply, the reformers put any and all feelings of sexual attraction, all desire, all passion not wholly motivated by the will to procreate, into the category of "burning."

So marriage was not, for the reformers, a place of proper bodily delight between a man and a woman. Rather, sex for pleasure even within marriage remained as much a sin as it had ever been in the Christian catalog. Moderation was their yardstick. "The *moderate* use of a woman in lawful matrimony," said Veron, was not sinful. Heinrich Bullinger expressed it even more strongly:

> Like as shamefastness, comeliness and temperance is good in everything, so it is good here also and exceeding necessary. Wedlock is honourable and holy, therefore must not we as shameless persons cast away good manners, and become like unreasonable beasts. God hath given and ordained marriage to be a remedy and medicine unto our feeble and weak flesh to swage the disquietness therefore, and to the intent that we should be clean and undefiled in spirit and in body. But if we rage therewith, and be shameless in words and deeds, then our mistemperance and excess may make it evil which is good and defile it that is clean.[9]

The ancient Christian distrust of physical passion and sensual abandonment remained as powerful as ever. Only William Tyndale seemed to offer an alternative view. "To take a wife for pleasure is as good as to abstain for displeasure," he wrote, defending the pleasures of marital sex with a forthrightness that is quite uncharacteristic of his time. Perhaps, however, his reasons were primarily polemical, for his defense of marital "pleasure" comes in his attack on the upholders of celibacy whom he characterises as being principally suspicious of marriage because of the sexual pleasure it provides.

For all that their arguments were based so solidly on Augustinian teaching, the reformers were at one critical point, however, revising the canon, though they did not often admit it. Augustine's "goods" of marriage did not include any provision of marital sex as remedy for sin. Peter Martyr, one of the more astute theologians among the reformers, was clear that remedy for sin was an additional "good" of marriage. Quoting Augustine that, within marriage, sex for procreation was reckoned to be without sin, he continued:

> Unto whose saying I have added this: that it must not be counted sin, when it happeneth to be done for avoiding of fornication.[10]

Martyr argues that the Church Fathers — such as Augustine — were in this instance overridden by the authority of Scripture. Note the legal metaphor Martyr uses. As for Augustine, similarly for the reformers: all sexual activity, even within marriage and even for procreation, was inherently sinful and defiling. But the *fact* of the marriage could "count" the sex act as sinless in certain circumstances. For Augustine, marriage was virtually for procreation only and for the artificial payment of the "debt"; for the reformers, it was also to be entered into for the avoidance of sin. Sex for sheer love or pleasure was "whorish, adulterous love" that was always and everywhere defiling.

With this circumscribed and suspicious view of human sexuality, it would have been unlikely for the reformers to see marriage as a desirable or positive way of life, one to be actively sought. On the contrary. To Parker, echoing John Colet in an earlier age, it was an indulgence to protect weak men from infirmity. To Martyr, marriage was not even to be sought as a redress for slight or occasional sexual urges. Rather, it was only for those struggling with temptations not to be borne, temptations so strong that

> we are not able to execute those things, which we ought to do; or else be so defiled, as we call not upon God with a good and pure conscience.[11]

This intolerable "burning" was in fact the means by which a man could understand that he was "called" to marriage. (The reformers were not interested in the sexual needs or concerns of women, except in so far as they were of service to men, a point to which we will return.)

Given this distasteful view of sexuality, it is not surprising that, with only a few notable exceptions, celibacy remained superior to marriage in the eyes of the Protestant reformers. They were at pains, however, to differentiate between what they defined as true celibacy and the "false" celibacy law of the Roman Catholic Church. True celibacy was a gift of God, something which could not be obtained by prayer, fasting or vows. The gift actually changed men's physical natures, eliminating sexual desire. It was an extremely rare gift, given by God to very few, and it was plain that striving to live single without having the gift was a waste of time. The reformers offered no substantial biblical exegesis to support this central claim, however.[12]

As celibacy was a gift, there was nothing meritorious in living a celibate life; this was beyond human power. Melanchthon explained that St Paul's praise of celibacy was simply praise for those who had the gift, as this meant they could the better serve God and the Church in their single state. While the unmarried life clearly was a more excellent state of life than that of the married, this, he argued was not a question of spiritual merit.[13] Martyr was adamant that "we be not of Jovinian's mind, that matrimony is to be accounted equal unto virginity." (Jovininian was the "heretic" whose views on the equal status of marriage prompted Augustine's famous rebuttal.) But Martyr insisted that this was so not because celibacy was intrinsically holier, but because "of the commodities and fewer causes of the distracting of the mind."[14]

Both Martyr and Martin Bucer claimed that men were actually predestined either to celibacy or to marriage. Just as God predestined his "elect" to eternal life, God also predestined the means by which they might reach eternity, said Martyr. Overwhelming sexual desire was thus a clear sign that a man was destined to marry rather than to live chaste. Prayer and "chastising the body" would "bring the flesh into subjection" in the case of the lesser temptations that a celibate could expect.[15] For Bucer, it was in the womb that God "fashioned" men for their calling, giving the gift of marriage as well as the gift of chastity. But, Bucer continued, though single life gave a man more freedom in the Lord's service, it was really but a minor consideration. If a man were as chaste "as a stone" but had "neither the study nor intelligence of Christ's kingdom," then he was a danger to the Church. He concluded tersely: "But that priests should only be without lawful wives, whom I pray you doth it profit a pin … ?'[16]

As celibacy could not be claimed to be superior because of spiritual merit, the reformers justified their theological preference on the basis that marriage was a burden. It was a distraction to the mind, a source of financial anxiety, and family cares. This was a useful point, as it enabled them to support their interpretation that St Paul's supposed preference for virginity (1 Corinthians 7:32–33) was based on the same argument and was not a matter of spiritual merit. This in turn protected them from falling foul of the doctrine of justification by faith alone in their admiration for chastity. For all their disclaimers, however, a lingering belief in celibacy as spiritually superior remains clearly discernible.

However, Thomas Becon – who quoted freely from Erasmus' lyrical praise of marriage – rejected any notion of marriage as being a heavy burden. He claimed much of this line of thought was traceable to the Roman Catholic Church's propaganda against marriage. He said, moreover, that in the cause of exalting celibacy, marriage's dignity had been "almost utterly defaced" – to the extent that it was labelled

> a kind of life base, unperfect, fleshly, troublesome, painful, unquiet, careful, unrestful, stuffed full of sorrow, calamity, misery, wretchedness, discord, strife, contention, debate … [17]

Becon preferred to see the married life as an opportunity for selfless love, in contrast to the self-centered ease of the single life.[18] But he remained a lone voice.

For the vast majority of the reformers, then, marriage was a necessary state of life and an indulgence to the weakness of most men who, without the gift of chastity, had to marry in order to control their fallen sexual drives. Sexual activity within marriage for this purpose, as well as for the procreation of children, was therefore acceptable, if regrettable. Though this is an extremely limited understanding of human sexuality from a modern perspective, it was at least a considerable advance on earlier theologies. It provided at last a justification for the relatively free exercise of sexual expression within marriage. Marital intercourse was neither unclean nor defiling. Nor should it be subject to any restraint other than the consciences of the couple concerned. Sex in marriage was given a new and radical legitimacy at last.

If this were the case, Barnes asked, could marriage defile prayers or contaminate sacrifices? Barnes was posing the central question of the marriage- celibacy debate of the sixteenth century. Could marriage be a holy way of life for the clergy? Yes, because did not St Paul prescribe marriage for the avoidance of fornication to "every" man (1 Corinthians 7:2)?[19] This was the crucial link in the reform doctrine of marriage and its application to the clergy. For to the reformers, the priest was the same as the layman in terms of his physical needs. If marriage was necessary for the control of sexual desires in fallen men, then it was necessary for *all* men, including the clergy. To exempt clergy from this precept of St Paul was, in effect, to demand of them "more articles of salvation ... than for princes or any other Christian men," as Barnes observed. Ordination neither takes away a man's "natural appetite" nor makes God's own remedy of marriage unlawful for the clergyman. Can ordination, Barnes asks, make unclean what is clean?[20]

Nowhere in these tracts is marriage commended to the clergy for loving companionship and support, for help in ministry, or for the joys of children and family life. It is promoted solely for the prevention of sexual sin, based on the premise that clergy are no different from other men, having the same physical needs and "infirmity." Ordination neither eases that infirmity nor changes the frail nature of men.

This in itself was a radical change. Through the Church's long tradition of exalting priestly celibacy can be traced the notion that clergy were a caste apart, differentiated in many ways from the laity. But in particular, their (theoretical) capacity to live the "angelic" life of virginity separated them as undeniably spiritually superior. For the reformers, however, the clergy were no different to other men, subject to the same weaknesses and temptations, requiring the same "remedies."

Their opponents, however, repeated the well-used arguments that insisted on priestly "purity" – which was narrowly defined in terms of cultic sexual abstinence: "He who stands at the altar must keep himself away from the sexual act." So, according to Christian tradition, sexual continence was demanded of priests because of their duties as celebrants of the Eucharist, as we have already seen. The reformers were usually less than adequate in their response to this powerful claim – a claim that still appears, explicitly, in twentieth-century Catholic teaching.[21]

Martyr, as might be expected, provided the most careful and thorough response. With a remarkably accurate understanding of the Jewish approach to bodily functions and ritual cleanliness, Martyr explained the origins of the Jewish taboos that had given an erroneous legitimacy to cultic purity claims in the Christian priesthood. Even in the "old law," he said, it cannot be proved that matrimonial intercourse made men "foul and unclean"; rather, the overriding Jewish fear was that of being contaminated with menstrual blood. For the Jews, it was physical uncleanness that defiled a man, but for Christians, it was sin. "Who is so far deceived as to say," Martyr asked, "that that disposition of the body [menstruation] is sin?" The Hebrew laws, then, required a separation from women on grounds that had no meaning at all in the Christian Church, as they dealt with a concept of uncleanness not to be equated with sinfulness. As sex within marriage for the sake of procreation or avoidance of sin was not itself sin, there was no basis for the traditional concept of priestly purity as sexual abstinence.[22]

There was, however, another side to this question of cultic purity. The special purity required of the priest was intimately linked to pre-reform doctrines of the Eucharist, such as transubstantiation and the sacrifice of the Mass. John Bale, always extreme and strident, nevertheless demonstrated graphically the nature of that connection:

> They said, that it was inconvenient, that he which has touched a woman should lay hands upon him, or admit him to office, that should make Christ's body ... where found these execrable hypocrites, that it was ever sin for a man to touch that vessel which was sanctified to his use? Either yet, where was power granted to their buggerish generation, to make Christ's body? ... Though in the Levitical priesthood they offered beasts, yet did not Christ leave it to thy massing priesthood to offer up his holy body and blood, thou traitorous massmonger. For he was able enough to offer up one effectual and perfect sacrifice for all.[23]

William Tyndale took the argument one step further, in a presentation of classic Protestant Eucharistic theology. The efficacy of the sacrament was dependent on the faith of the communicant; it only became the body and blood of Christ spiritually and individually, he insisted. There was no more need for the man who said Mass or ministered it to be any purer than those who heard it or received it. Besides, even if Christ were physically present in the Mass, he could not be defiled by any man's hands, "be they never so unwashed."[24]

And yet, the ancient taboo still lingered behind the relentless logic of their arguments. Martyr, so powerful in his intellectual precision – the clearest exponent of the sinlessness of marital sexual activity – nevertheless recommended that both clergy and laity should refrain from sex for short times, particularly when the sacraments were to be administered or received, "so that the conscience persuade hereunto, that it may be done without breach of charity." The clergy, in fact, should refrain "oftener than other men."[25] Melanchthon asserted that "godly men know when and how long the conjugal act should be moderated and restrained."[26]

These recommendations for occasional cultic abstinence are a telling indicator of the profound struggle in which these men were personally involved. In the same way, their continuing insistence on the superiority of virginity alerts us to the reality that the reformers had not shaken off the old paradigm. All of them had been educated in the old thought-world; they had been ordained under the old dispensation. Some had been monks. Even as they strove to build a coherent argument for clerical marriage, they were unable to divorce it from the prevailing tradition. So the reasons they offered for the acceptability of clerical marriage were not born of a new understanding of sex and marriage at all; rather, as we have seen, they adapted the old understanding to fit their case. Celibacy was still honored, though with a different theological base; the sex drive was still primarily a disease, though a disease that could be controlled – not through celibacy, but through marriage.

Perhaps the most significant change in their theology in terms of clergy marriage was that the priest no longer had a cultic role that demanded sexual purity. The changed understanding of the Eucharist clearly lay behind that. But was there in fact a changed notion of priestly purity also at work behind their intellectual wrestlings?

One of the major arguments the reformers offered for clerical marriage was straightforward and practical. Quite simply, the celibacy law was not working. For all the protestations that celibacy was the only acceptable lifestyle for clergy, the reformers claimed most clergy were not in fact living chaste lives. John Bale's *Acts of English Votaries* was a lurid and sensational catalog of stories of clerical immorality performed under the guise of celibacy, but the more restrained reformers also referred to the loose living of the supposedly celibate clergy of Rome. Barnes maintained that only one-third of the English clergy kept their chastity, a fact he claimed was well known to the Church. Historians have questioned the accuracy of these claims, maintaining that they were grossly exaggerated for polemical purposes. They may well have been. But it is worth remembering that John Colet, the austere priest of the pre-Reformation period who had nothing to do with the Protestant schism or its debate, made similar claims about clerical immorality.[27] Modern observers know only too well that Roman Catholic clergy continue to suffer lapses from their vows, and that in some parts of the world de facto relationships are common. The recent evidence of large-scale sexual abuse perpetrated on both women and minors by Roman Catholic priests and brothers is unlikely to be a historical aberration, demonstrating as it does the unsuitability of compulsory celibacy for many people. It is unlikely that the situation in the sixteenth century was very different.

What distressed the reformers – and the level of their distress is evident through their prose – was the hypocrisy that lay behind the claims made for celibacy. Here were clergy living manifestly immoral lives under the guise of celibacy, but priests who had married were the ones declared to be immoral. "Is then a whore's flesh clean that priests may handle it while that of an honest and good woman is not?" asked Barnes. "What hath pure matrimony offended, that it alonely [sic] should defile priests' hands, and all other manner of vices, and uncleanness, doth nothing contaminate them?" Bale suggests it is a strange kind of chastity that is "every week polluted": "Yet may they after this learning, every day say mass, their vow never hindered, but in marriage they may not so … "[28]

The "Pope's shavelings," wrote Veron, say it is less offence for them to lie with "a hundred harlots, than to have wives of their own." They claim they can the next day repent and be shriven, obtaining from the pope's hands free remission of their sins. But if they married, they would live "in continual uncleanliness, and stinking pollution, whereby ... we shall never be pure and clean, for to come to the altar of the Lord."[29] Marriage is thus considered a continual and unforgivable defilement, while sexual immorality can always be ritually absolved, allowing even the most debauched priest to fulfil the Church's cultic requirements. Marriage involved a fundamental changing of the rules, while extramarital sexual activity merely broke the rules. The modern dilemma in the Catholic Church over the celibacy law, and in all the mainstream churches over the ordination of practicing homosexuals, has some interesting parallels with the situation that the reformers faced. This is an issue to which we will return.

In this question of priestly purity lay the crux of the whole debate for the reformers; the question turned on the distinction between holiness of life and ritual holiness, and the relationship these different attitudes bore to the traditional and reformed understandings of the priesthood. The reformers, who had abandoned a cultic model of ministry, were not interested in a cultically pure priesthood. They needed a model of priesthood that offered a standard of moral living for wider society.

Central to the Reformation was the place of preaching. Gone was the centrality of the sacraments, and particularly that of the Eucharist. Instead, the word of God and its exposition was exalted to such a degree that, in time, the Bible would be called the "paper pope." Again and again, the reformers we have been studying equated true ministry with the "pure preaching of the Gospel." Bale asked what sort of religion it was that "was all to do with praying and not preaching, singing and not feeding the flock, cleansing by outward ceremonies and not by inward faith?"[30] Rituals of the senses had given way to a cerebral ritual of words.

The Protestant reformers did not invent the art of preaching, but they placed it at the heart of Christian ministry. The relationship between preaching's new role and that of clerical marriage was clear-cut. For preaching to be truly effective, the reformers believed, the preacher had to practice what he preached. It was no use preaching about holiness of life if the preacher himself lived scandalously. Tyndale summarized this point succinctly:

> the people look as well unto the living as unto the preaching, and are hurt at once if the living disagree, and fall from the faith, and believe not the word.[31]

In fact, the lifestyle of the clergy was a living sermon for common people, and "most of all unto the weakest," for whom the priest should be "endued with all virtue and honesty." Tellingly, Tyndale says that the chastity of wives, daughters, and servants is of great concern to ordinary men, against whom the "unchaste chastity of the spirituality" is a grave danger. The open moral integrity of the clergy clearly had implications for the well-being of the wider society.[32]

The first Anglican Ordinal of 1550 enshrined this concern for the personal morality of the clergyman and his family, and pointed to the teaching value of the example set. The service of Ordering of Priests included an exhortation to the candidates that required them to be "wholesome and godly examples and patterns" for the rest of the congregation to follow. Their calling was such that they must take care neither to "offend" God in their own lives nor to be "occasion that other offend." In this exhortation the "teaching-office and personal life of the priest are didactically emphasised as they had not been in the Latin rite," F. E. Brightman, an early commentator on the prayer book, has pointed out.

The eight questions the bishop then publicly asked the candidates underscored the priest's role as moral exemplar, expressed thus:

> Will you be diligent to frame and fashion your own selves, and your families, according to the doctrine of Christ, and to make both yourselves and them (as much as in you lieth) wholesome examples and spectacles to the flock of Christ?

Like the exhortation, these questions have no parallel in the Latin rites; instead, they are very similar to Bucer's rite of ordination, and scholars are divided over which came first. Every succeeding Ordinal, to the present day, repeated this Ordination emphasis on the clerical family as a model for the community. The Ordinal's overall emphasis on teaching and guiding, rather than the cultic or ceremonial role of the clergy, encapsulates the reform understanding of priesthood that informed the specific issue of clerical marriage.[33]

The reformers' concern for the moral health of the laity, which stood behind this marriage model, was not merely a matter of the general good of the society, though that was important to them. Their aim was to create a "godly" society which, in their terms, could only come about when individuals lived godly lives. Their overriding concern was for individual salvation, an urgent issue now that the former ritual modes of achieving purity in the eyes of God had been discredited. Despite the reformers' theological reliance on the doctrine of justification by faith alone, the corpus of their beliefs in fact required adherence to a strict ethical and moral standard in personal life. With the practice of confession, the sacrifice of the Mass, and the notion of sacramental grace all condemned, lay people and clergy alike had nothing else to rely on but their own personal purity. There was, in the reformers' scenario, little room for mistake or change in any individual. As the Ordinal put it, the chief end of the priests' ministry was to bring their congregations to such a level of faith, knowledge, and spiritual development that there would be no room in them either for "error in religion, or for viciousness in life." The image is one of a relentless upward spiral of spiritual growth, leading to a pattern of uniformity in both Church and society.

Reformation teaching had revived the long-dormant understanding of the "priesthood of all believers," and the reformers stressed the importance for the clergy of teaching their flocks how to share in that priestliness. Implicit in this understanding was the notion that the clergyman's role differed from the lay person's in degree rather than kind. The laity were bound by the Gospel to pray as much as priests were, insisted Barnes; and Bale argued that the commitment accepted by the priest at ordination was essentially no different to the Christian commitment of any lay person, regardless of age, sex, or status. For Ponet, priests were no holier than lay people, though the celibacy rule had created in the people a false impression of the clergy. It gave them an "opinion of holiness … for that they married not as other men did." The clergy themselves had been blinded by the "gain they got by their unworthy estimation."[34]

Certainly, the exaltation of celibacy for the clergy could not have helped lay people esteem marriage as a holy way of life. In his strenuous defense of celibacy written in 1554, Thomas Martin described marriage as "the basest state of life in Christ's Church," for sexual desire was of the devil. Marital sexual activity, he maintained, was always unclean, even if lawful.[35] Melanchthon recognized the harm that such teaching did to married people, who could not but doubt that "their acts of wedlock and duties of matrimony" displeased God.[36] So priestly marriage, for the reformers, was a means of promoting and encouraging marriage among the laity. The reformers' task was to make marriage unequivocally a "holy estate."

Thomas Cranmer's famous preamble to the marriage service in the Book of Common Prayer summed up this attitude. Marriage was an "honourable estate," a "holy estate," "commended of St Paul to be honourable among all men." He outlined three "causes" for which matrimony had been ordained: first, for procreation; second, as a "remedy against sin, and to avoid fornication: that such persons as have not the gift of continency might marry, and keep themselves undefiled members of Christ's body"; and third, for the "mutual society, help, and comfort, that the one ought to have of the other." Modern Anglican services have modernized this line in order to suggest that marriage must be honored *by* all, but almost certainly Cranmer meant more than that. In the light of the contemporary struggle for priestly marriage, there can be little doubt that he meant that it was a way of life honorable *for* all men, including clergy. His very marriage service was part of the progaganda, not least because of its radical listing of "remedy against sin" as one of the "causes." And did Cranmer, or his liturgical predecessor, have in mind the then recent enforced separation of priests and their wives when he incorporated the Matthean sentence, "Those whom God hath joined together: let no man put asunder" (Matthew 19:6), immediately before the official pronouncement of marriage?[37]

The concern for promoting marriage in the wider community through the example of a married clergy was part of a broader campaign against immorality that grew apace during the second half of the sixteenth century. The Protestant Reformation brought a growing demand for the introduction of harsher penalties against sexual offenders. In part, the zeal of the reformers in this area was motivated by their fierce opposition to the Church of Rome, in this case prompted by their belief that the Roman Catholic Church took a far too lenient view of sexual immorality. This was evident in the behavior of their own clergy, which had in turn promoted the general acceptance of lax moral standards in the community. The official Church of England homily against whoredom complained that this vice was not regarded as a sin, but more as a "pastime, a dalliance."

In the first days of the formal English Reformation, under Edward VI, the ill-fated *Reformatio Legum Ecclesiasticarum* contained ferocious sanctions for sexual offenses. This English revision of church laws was brought to Parliament in March 1553, but the death of the young king shortly afterwards caused it to lapse. Later Protestants brought a series of bills to Parliament which, if implemented, would have brought severe penalties for adultery, fornication, and bastardy. These foundered, in part because many members of parliament feared that "men of quality might be subjected to 'base' punishments for sexual transgressions"![38]

The only laws passed, in the end, were acts against illegitimacy in 1576 and 1610 which, while they fell far short of the demands of the more vociferous churchmen, still represented a hardening of the law against sexual offenders. It is worth remembering, however, that in the growing poverty of the lower classes in the later Elizabethan period, adultery and fornication could lead to heavy costs on individual parishes, which were burdened with the support of illegitimate children. The moral outrage of clergy and government reflected the need to find answers to a significant economic problem. It is interesting that their attitude to sexual activity during betrothal was generally ambivalent, which suggests that it was casual sexual activity without commitment or obligation, rather than sex before marriage *per se*, that was the object of their primary concern, not least because of its financial costs to the community.[39]

The exaltation of *marriage*, not chastity, had become the new and practical means to the creation of a godly society. To spearhead that development, a new kind of priestly purity was essential. The celibate model had manifestly not worked – not for the clergy and not, because of the poor example they set, for the society that they served. The new priestly purity, based on a strict and enduring commitment to a particular moral standard, required a married clergy able, through their marriage, to control the destructive sexual drive in a way that was similarly possible for all lay people. It was a radical turning of the tables on nearly 1500 years of Christian teaching, made possible only by a new Eucharistic theology that no longer required the ritual purity of sexual abstinence. It could, however, be argued that the new purity was, in its own way, just as "cultic" as the old. The whole "godly society" became a separate caste.

The Protestant reformers' exaltation of marriage was still a long way from being a warm affirmation of human sexuality, let alone a celebration of sexual love and affection. It was almost mechanical, a means to an end. And it remained hedged about by all the distrust and suspicion that had accompanied the ancient taboo. That taboo had still not been challenged directly; rather, it had been nibbled around the edges, leaving the central doctrine of the superiority of sexual abstinence firmly intact, if diminished in practical terms. Given the context of the reformers' struggle, their own origins, and the backgrounds of the people they sought to convince, this is not surprising, however disappointing it might be for modern minds.

Clerical marriage was the practical and unmistakable expression of many Reformation doctrines. First and foremost, married priests proclaimed a new order of priesthood more effectively than any amount of theological discourse alone, a priesthood that was both radically different from the cultic priestly caste of the Roman Catholic Church and integral to a new sacramental theology. Married clergy were members of the priesthood of all believers, not the heirs of the Aaronic priesthood. They offered no sacrifice, and did not mediate between God and God's people. Their role in presiding at the Holy Communion required no special holiness. Rather, they were ministers whose primary role was to exhort and encourage lay people to a holiness of life that expressed itself primarily in a rigid personal moral uprightness, thus creating a reformed and godly society. By implication, it proclaimed a new Church.

This was a practical demonstration of the key Reformation doctrine of Justification by faith alone; there was no longer any merit in denying the sexual urge and striving to live a life of angelic perfection. In this way, the reformed priesthood demonstrated the reality of fallen human nature and the consequent dependence on the mercy of God through clerical acceptance of the "remedy" God had provided for human weakness.

Nevertheless, whether or not they realized it, the reformers were agents in what can only be called a paradigm shift. The ambiguities within their arguments, and the existence of the occasional lone voice overthrowing the old order in one area or another, bear witness to that. One such voice was that of Martin Bucer. Bucer – one of the first Continental reformers to marry – grounded his doctrine of marriage in the doctrine of predestination. Some were called to marriage, some to celibacy, he said. Both states of life were holy for those called into them. Marriage was primarily ordained neither for the sake of procreation nor to offer a remedy for sin. Alone among the reformers, Bucer consistently claimed that the first cause, or reason, for marriage was mutual society and support. The care and love of husband and wife, and the bearing and raising of children, Bucer claimed, were not simply worldly activities – let alone a distracting burden – but were in fact celestial. The full articulation of this understanding of marriage can be found in the commentary he wrote on the 1549 Book of Common Prayer. Criticizing the priorities given there for marriage – children first, remedy for sin second, mutual society third – he wrote:

> I should prefer that what is placed third among the causes of marriage might be in the first place, because it is first. For a true marriage can take place between people who seek neither for children nor for a remedy against fornication … yet since the "two are one flesh" and live unto God as one person, it follows that without that union of minds and bodies and possessions by which the husband shows himself to be the head of the wife and the wife a helper of her husband for every purpose of godly and holy living it is no true and real marriage before God.[40]

Overlooking his commitment to male headship, Bucer's view of marriage as a joyful union not necessarily dedicated to overcoming sin is surprisingly close to modern theological understandings of marriage, as reflected in the most recent marriage liturgies.[41] But it has taken more than 400 years for the Anglican Church to accept his ordering, and all that it implies.

The reformers' commitment to a married clergy heralded a changing theology of marriage. In itself, that embryonic theology would certainly not have been sufficiently powerful an impetus for this radical change in Church order without there being the overriding commitment to a new model of priesthood. Without the reformers' realizing it, however, the arguments for and the reality of a married priesthood gave a substantial boost to changes in thought about sex and marriage that were already beginning to form. The fact that the community's moral and religious leaders could at last marry without detriment to their calling marked a crucial stage on the path to the revolution of ideas that in later years would see marriage become a positive rather than a negative means to holiness. This, at least in theory, would overturn completely the ancient preference for asceticism.

6

PRODDING THE
CHURCH TO CHANGE ■

The Roman Catholic Church did not follow the lead of the Protestant and Anglican Churches in allowing clergy to marry. To this day, the issue remains a pressing one. In recent decades in particular – since the wide-ranging changes of the Second Vatican Council freed the clergy in many areas – there has been an almost constant pressure for change in this area, too, but so far to no avail. As a direct consequence, there is a serious world-wide shortage of priests, attributed to the Church's failure to permit a married clergy. Not only have many clergy left the priesthood to marry, but many potential ordinands in recent times have been unwilling to commit themselves to the celibate ideal.

In the decades immediately following the Protestant schism, however, there were various attempts to open up the celibacy debate within the Catholic Church. Some of the princely leaders of European states that had remained Catholic argued for the introduction of a married clergy as one way to counter the devastating effects of the Reformation. But the Council of Trent, the Church's eighteen-year, exhaustive counter-response to the Reform movement, did not even deal with the subject until its closing sessions.

At its second last session, in 1563, the council revealed its mind. It declared as "anathema" any who claimed that clerical marriage was valid. It was only the fact that the Eastern Church continued to allow a married clergy that prevented the council from declaring celibacy a "divine" rather than an "ecclesiastical" law. Ironically, this reponse to the Reformation actually hardened the Church against clerical marriage, and led to an even stronger defense of the celibate life.

But the council went further. It also condemned any who suggested that marriage was better than, or even on a par with, virginity and celibacy. The ancient spiritual superiority of these two virtues was powerfully reinforced. In the Catechism based on the decrees of Trent, the age-old preference for sexual abstinence, or at the very least sexual moderation, was once again promoted to the faithful. In particular, several "questions" in the Catechism spelt out the need for married couples to restrain their sexual activities to procreation and "remedy." Question 33 makes plain that "marriage is not to be used from motives of sensuality or pleasure." It quotes Jerome:

> A wise man … ought to love his wife with judgement, not with the impulse of passion … there is no greater turpitude than that a husband should love his wife as he would an adulteress.[1]

In passing, it is interesting to note, however, that the Roman Catholic Church had adopted "remedy" as one of the reasons for marriage and sexual activity within it. This, as we have seen, was not one of the "causes" promoted by Augustine of Hippo or by any of the mainstream pre-Reformation theologians. It was the reformers who gave it prominence yet, within so short a time, it had slipped virtually unnoticed into Roman teaching as well. In the same way, over the following centuries the Church of Rome would follow the Protestants in adopting a more positive view of sex and marriage. The heritage is not only unacknowledged, but actually unnoticed!

In their own time, however, the reformers' promotion of marriage met with limited currency in the Western world. The bulwark of Rome stood firm as ever. And even in Protestant countries the long shadows of asceticism retreated only slowly. There was no sudden change in the attitudes of Protestants to sex and marriage, even with the model of a married priesthood before them. It has been pointed out that "advice to the married" in fact changed little before and after the Reformation, so that Trent's teaching against sexual enjoyment within marriage would have been quite acceptable among most Protestants.[2] It was not until considerably later that sex and marriage attained the quasi-sacred status they hold in Protestant (and Catholic) teaching. Paradigms shift slowly.

In passing it is worth mentioning that, uniquely among the reformed churches, the Anglican Church – particularly in its High Church and Anglo-Catholic expressions – has retained a respect for celibacy. Unlike other Protestant churches, it has been happy for its clergy to remain unmarried, should they so choose. This, however, has meant that the notion that celibacy is a higher ideal than marriage has survived in some quarters. Earlier this century, an English priest, Edward Maycock, composed a sad and telling prayer:

> Forgive me Lord for thinking years ago that to serve
> you as a priest unmarried was service of a higher,
> better kind;
> That love, the greatest of your gifts to man, was best
> sublimated, not expressed;
> That marriage, with responsibility for family life, was a
> lower form of priestly service.
> And now that years have passed, help me to bear the
> burden of the consequence, the burden of loving and
> longing to love more, yet bound by no gesture to
> indicate that love to those beloved.[3]

In the late-sixteenth and early-seventeenth centuries, one of the most significant developments that arose from the clerical marriage controversy was voiced by some radical Puritans in England. They argued for a shift in emphasis on marriage; for them, the role of marriage was primarily for mutual society and comfort, for affection, and, ideally, for the "marriage of true minds." This brought marriage doctrine much closer to modern notions, and was a significant development in some quarters in that it led to a reconsideration of the permissible grounds for divorce, an issue to which we will return. But again, it remained strangely cut off from a changed understanding of sexuality. Though there were some who actually celebrated the sexual component of married life, most remained theoretically constrained by the thought-world of Jerome. Love in marriage was almost entirely separate from sexual activity, which was never depicted as an expression of conjugal love. Sex remained a physical appetite to be controlled rather than a joyous act of bodily communion. In fact, the ideal of married love was that a man should love his wife "as a sister," not as a whore. It is telling that until relatively recent times there was no concept of anything in between these extremes.

Closely connected with this failure to discern the potential of marriage to be a genuinely mutual sexual partnership was the view of women that underscored the theology of the reformers and their immediate heirs. Their view is readily summed up in their favorite euphemism for sex: "the use of the woman." Again and again, this is their euphemism for sexual intercourse. In this context, women are seen as little more than sex aids for providing relief for male urges. Barnes and Bale both referred to wives as "vessels" who were owned by men for their legitimate use, while Tyndale wrote that women were created for men's necessity and "therefore a man may use her at all his need in all degrees."[4]

As men of their time, the reformers subscribed to the commonly held Aristotelian view of woman as a faulty creation. Women were not only misbegotten; their faultiness had been increased by the Fall to a far greater degree than that which prevailed in men. Martyr was explicit:

> Even when nature was uncorrupted, seeing woman was more unperfect than man, she should after a sort have been ruled by him: for she was made for him, and to be a help unto him. But when sin had now corrupted our nature, the imperfection of woman was grievously

sed; and therefore she had need to be more
ly ruled by man.[5]

But some of the reformers – even while clearly holding to the traditional theological view of women's inferiority – were concerned that women should not be despised, as women were by many of those who promoted celibacy. Bale identifies strong anti-women feeling among those who exalted celibacy: "So perverse stomachs have they borne to women, that the more part of their tempting spirits they have made she devils."

He relates stories of saints "who had so great malice unto women" that they plagued women with illness if they presumed to come to their shrines. He also recognized that the belief that marriage rendered a man cultically impure was based not so much on male sexuality as on the fact that it involved a physical relationship with a woman. Nevertheless, Bale was no proto-feminist. He was quick to deride women at the suggestion that there was any comparison between female vows of chastity and priests' vows of celibacy:

> ... they are brought to a narrow shift, that seeketh to be
> holpen by women's matters. What hath widowhood to
> do with priesthood, more than womanhood with
> massing? Are the offices of priest and woman become
> now all one? Then let priests be women also ... [6]

Melanchthon linked the anti-women attitude prevalent among many Roman writers with their degraded views of marriage,[7] and so hinted at one of the unplanned benefits of clergy marriage. If marriage is portrayed as a good and holy state of life, then there has to be at least some degree of respect for both partners within it. The doctrine of women's inferiority has to be modified so that it does not jeopardize this high view. Similarly, if priests can marry, then women by extension can no longer be depicted as defiling. Nor can women any longer be identified as temptresses, leading men into sin, if they are the means by which men are saved from sin. A married priesthood encouraged a higher view of women than had previously been the case.

Some feminists have argued that the Reformation actually diminished the role of women by closing religious orders that had at least offered a tiny number of upper-class women some measure of educational and professional opportunity. While this may be true, it ignores the heightened level of respect married women gained through the abolition of the celibacy law. Before the Reformation, women vowed to virginity were the only women to receive any real measure of respect within the Church. In the reformed churches, through the new phenomenon of a married clergy, married women – women who did not deny their sexual and bodily functions – gained a new status.

Ironically, clergy wives were themselves caught between the two ideals. In polemical Protestant literature, they enjoyed the high estimation paid to the "godly matron," though the protagonists of clerical marriage gave surprisingly little thought to the role of the vicarage wife. Joye, writing under the name of Sawtry, drew up a formidable job description that expected the ideal clergy wife to be "sober, learned, modest, shamefaced, simple, sad, chaste," but also only too willing to tackle the most menial household chores as well as to visit the sick and poor, "be they never so lothely."[8] But in the wider community, where the old prejudices against the women who consorted with priests remained strong, clergy wives often faced continuing revulsion. Even as late as the early-nineteenth century, clergy were considered poor matches for well-born women, though by then the main concern was their low income rather than social status. Jane Austen's novels offer excellent examples of this prejudice! It would take until the late-Victorian era, with its growing emphasis on rigid moral standards, before the clergy wife would become the paragon of virtue of the Trollope novels.

One of the immediate outcomes of the Reformation debate about marriage was a reconsideration of the grounds of divorce. From the earliest days of the Reformation, there can be traced a minority view that the first "cause" of marriage was companionship ("mutual society") rather than either procreation, which had always dominated traditional Christian theology, or remedy, so strongly promoted by the reformers. The Strasbourg reformer Martin Bucer, as we have seen, took issue with Cranmer's marriage service published in the first Book of Common Prayer of 1549. Bucer argued that priority should have been given to mutual society.[9]

Cranmer ignored Bucer's suggestion. In all subsequent editions of the Book of Common Prayer, procreation and remedy retained their priority over mutual society. This rigid order has been diluted only in recent times. Contemporary Australian Anglican liturgies in fact place procreation as the third "cause" of matrimony – a little-noticed radical reversal of the traditional position.[10]

This Anglican refusal to jettison the traditional understanding of marriage, despite the lengthy clerical marriage debate, in part explains that church's long objection to divorce. It indicates, too, the triumph of continuity of doctrine over the more radical aspects of reformed thinking, despite considerable Puritan influence on the fledgling Church of England in the sixteenth and early-seventeenth centuries.

Puritan writers were strong advocates of the importance of the total relationship in marriage. They regarded mutual love, and a high level of intellectual and emotional compatibility, as primary to a real marriage. So marriage for them was first and foremost a covenant between two people rather than a sacramental relationship imposed by God's action. For most Puritans, this covenant relationship was just as binding, just as indissoluble, as a sacramental one. But for a minority – including Bucer and later the English poet John Milton – it opened the way to divorce. If the mutuality died, then so did the marriage.[11]

However, few reformers took so radical a view. Mainstream Continental reformers did allow for the dissolution of a marriage on grounds of unfaithfulness or desertion, and sometimes of impotence. Some reformed churches, such as the church in Geneva, were stricter than others, for example that in Scotland, in their interpretation of basically the same principles. Only the

Church of England, among all the reformed churches, retained the Roman Catholic concept of total indissolubility.

This is, at first glance, ironic, given the marital adventures of Henry VIII, who was responsible for the formation of the Church of England as a separate entity. However, he exploited the concept of annulment – the notion that no true marriage had been validly entered – to end three of his six marriages. The preeminent historian of divorce, Roderick Phillips, believes that Henry's refusal to contemplate divorce as an option actually established the anti-divorce stance of the Church of England for the next 300 years.

The Church of England did, however, flirt with divorce in its first attempt at writing its own set of canon law. The *Reformatio Legum Ecclesiasticarum*, devised by a commission of bishops, theologians and lawyers during the reign of Edward VI, provided for divorce on several grounds, including adultery, desertion, prolonged absence without news, and attempted murder. The *Reformatio*, however, died with Edward VI. When the definitive Canons of 1604 were formulated half a century later, the climate had changed. While separation was possible, divorce was explicitly ruled out. The Church of England remained firmly wedded to the rules of the Church of Rome on this matter.

But in so doing, Anglicans were not committing themselves to an undeviating pattern of Christian teaching! On the contrary, they were holding to a more recent pattern, introduced by the same Gregorian popes who had ruled so harshly against clerical marriage. The tightening of the Church's position against divorce happened only in the eleventh and twelfth centuries, while the utter indissolubility of marriage as church law dates only from the thirteenth century. The early Church had been quite ambivalent about divorce and remarriage, and this continued into the early medieval period. Adultery, however, was generally the only permissible grounds for divorce, and was available only for the wronged husband.

Adultery remained the sole grounds for divorce until relatively recent times. As Phillips points out, the adultery of a wife was always regarded far more seriously than that of a husband, and was the matrimonial offence *par excellence*. This was directly linked to procreation as the primary cause of marriage: if a woman committed adultery the husband lost the certainty of paternity of the sons who would inherit his property and name. The adultery of the husband was relatively unimportant, because the offense was one of property rather than of sexual propriety or even trust. This was in keeping with ancient marital laws. Theologians have demonstrated the overriding principle of protection of property obtaining in Judaic rules against adultery.[12]

The reformers, despite their often radical revision of marriage doctrine, were unable to shake off the concept of the indissolubility of marriage. Their theology and, indeed, their experience of being the first lawfully married theologians in many centuries drove them to adopt what Phillips has called a higher estimation of marriage than the Church of Rome. They were, he argues, concerned more with the content of the marriage, the quality of the marital relationship, than with the form:

> In the sixteenth century the Protestants were groping towards a broader conception of marriage than Catholic doctrines and laws had permitted ... But they were still too close to the breach with Rome to be able to shed entirely the unease inspired by the conclusions about divorce to which the logic of their social theology drove them.[13]

In a similar way, as we have seen, they held back from the logical conclusions of their theological explorations of human sexuality and the marital relationship.

One of the factors that inhibited the emergence of a more liberal attitude toward divorce was the centrality of the family unit to society in the seventeenth century. The same theologians who struggled with theological concepts of divorce were also lyrical in their praise of the family as the guarantor of social and political order. Marriage breakdown posed an unacceptable danger to this order, and not only in the seventeenth century.

Phillips identifies this factor as perhaps the major reason accounting for why the demand for divorce continued to be so rare until the modern period. Marriage breakdown in traditional European society was almost inconceivable for most people, because the family unit was integral to the economy. Husbands and wives learned to live together despite adultery, violence, abuse, and other difficulties because life as a separated person was far more difficult than life within marriage. Family members were interdependent in pre-industrial society; a person on their own was highly vulnerable. This was particularly so for a woman, whose economic plight could be desperate if she were deserted or even widowed. Rapid rates of remarriage after widowhood testify to the urgent need to restore the protection of the family unit.[14]

Phillips argues that it is wrong to place the blame for modern rates of divorce on a high level of instability in marriage relationships *per se*. Rather, they reflect the substantial changes that have occurred in the social, economic, and demographic contexts of marriage. As industrialization and urbanization revolutionized European society, opportunities for life outside marriage increased. So the level of tolerance dropped. Husbands and wives no longer had to tolerate the intolerable in a way that earlier generations did. A corresponding demand for divorce and remarriage was inevitable.

There had, of course, been earlier demands for divorce and remarriage, principally among the upper classes, for whom the social and economic consequences were minimal. Because church law resolutely opposed any form of divorce, the first formal divorces in Protestant England had to be gained through the back door. In 1669, John Manners, Lord Roos, introduced a private member's bill into Parliament in order to secure his divorce, so that he could remarry and father an heir. He was already separated from his wife on the grounds of her adultery.

Others took up the precedent, but the numbers remained small. Divorce by private member's bill was a costly, complex process, available only to the wealthy. First, the couple had to be granted a formal separation by a church court. Next, the aggrieved husband (adultery was the only grounds for parliamentary divorce) needed to exact financial compensation from his wife's lover (for he had been deprived of his property) before parliamentary dissolution could be granted. From 1670 to 1857, only 325 divorces were achieved by this means – one or two per year. Only four divorces were granted to women, who had to prove aggravated adultery – adultery compounded by incest or bigamy. It took until 1923 before English women were given equal access to divorce on grounds of simple adultery – a manifest example of the sexual "double standard" at work, and undeniable evidence that for most of Christian history adultery has been condemned principally because it damaged a man's property rights. Women, having no such rights, had no recourse against their husband's adultery unless it was "aggravated."[15] The enormity of the hypocrisy that lay behind the solemn rhetoric of church leaders over the centuries on the adultery question is staggering to the modern mind: male property rights were protected under the guise of upholding a rigid sexual propriety that was, nevertheless, completely one-sided!

By the early-nineteenth century, with England now urbanized and industrialized, the demand for greater access to divorce was rising. The state's assumption of control over marriage in the 1753 *Hardwicke Act* had begun the process of disengaging marriage law from the Church. But the Church remained bitterly opposed to any greater access to divorce and particularly to remarriage. In 1800, the Bishop of London spoke against attempts to allow a woman who had been divorced on grounds of adultery to remarry. This, he said, would only give her a "reward for her misconduct."[16]

In 1857, the first English divorce law was passed by Parliament. The grounds were still only adultery for husbands, aggravated adultery for wives. But at least the lengthy procedure of the private member's bill was now obsolete. The Church of England, however, in common with the Roman Catholic Church, continued to oppose divorce implacably. In the 1870s, the Anglican Church tried to ban any form of remarriage in church after divorce, though an 1885 committee of bishops suggested a more liberal stance. The church should remarry innocent parties, it said, and even perhaps repentant guilty parties having episcopal approval. The 1888 Lambeth Conference – the meeting of Anglican bishops from the worldwide Anglican Communion – recommended allowing the innocent party remarriage in church and access to the sacraments. Given that women were still required to prove "aggravated adultery" to instigate a divorce action, this meant that the vast majority of "innocent" parties were, of course, men.

A survey of the English dioceses in the 1890s revealed different rules operating in different places. Divorced people who wished to remarry in church needed only to find a sympathetic diocese. But given the strict residency requirements for marriages at the time, this would not have been as easy as it might seem, particularly in a less mobile society.[17]

In Australia, the Anglican Church showed a similar reluctance to permit divorce and remarriage. In New South Wales in 1887, that church was instrumental in holding up the liberalization of divorce law. The New South Wales Parliament wanted to add desertion, assault, drunkenness, and long-term imprisonment as grounds for divorce, but provoked a storm of opposition that was whipped up by the Sydney Anglican synod. In the end, the Bishop of Sydney, Bishop Alfred Barry, petitioned Queen Victoria to withhold her approval. It took until 1892 for her assent to be given.[18]

In passing, it is interesting to note the double standard at work here. The clergy were presumably not directly aware that they were complicit in continuing a grave injustice. Adultery was clearly the grounds for divorce most necessary for married men if they felt humiliated by their wives' behavior and by the threat to their paternity and property. However, the new grounds for divorce in New South Wales were grounds most needed by women, who were most at risk from desertion, assault, drunkenness, and imprisonment. These circumstances were potentially far more threatening for them than their husbands' sexual infidelity could ever be. This signals powerfully the churches' masculine bias and one-eyed approach on issues of sexuality. It betrays, too, an ugly hypocrisy: the use of twisted theological reasoning in order to justify the dissolution of a marriage if a man's property rights were threatened but not if a woman's very life was put at risk.

Sir Alfred Stephen, the framer of the New South Wales Divorce Extension Bill and an upholder of Christian values, was himself motivated by the suffering of many families at the hands of violent men. He condemned church leaders for their narrow and literalist use of Scripture in their arguing against a more humane solution to these very real problems. But as Sydney historian Dr Bill Lawton has pointed out, church leaders saw this move as just one more nail in the coffin of the Church's domination of society. They were fearful that, as was the case when the ancient prohibition against marrying a deceased wife's sister ended, they were witnessing the thin end of the wedge. Humanist anti-Christian, even anti-British, forces were at work, they feared, and the kingdom of God was under siege. Their arguments, however, found no favor with wider society, where they were condemned for the narrowness of their views and their lack of charity. Dr Lawton states that the Sydney clergy were obsessed by semantics; in full flight from the "secularist bogey," they had no other place to hide. The protest was out of step, not only with public opinion generally, but with that of the majority of churchgoers.[19]

Dr Lawton points to a general Anglican reactionary stance that existed at the time and no doubt helped retard the Church's response to urgent community problems for decades. The formation, in Australia in 1892, of the Mothers' Union, a conservative association designed to exalt the role of the mother in upholding traditional family values, was perhaps the longest-lasting influence. With branches in nearly every parish, it romanticized the purity of womanhood and elevated the concept of the duty of the wife and mother. It stood firmly against growing notions of female independence and autonomy, and even objected to giving women the vote.[20] (How far it helped to retard the Church's response to calls for women in the priesthood throughout this century can only be guessed at.) While it admitted single women to membership, it firmly denied the same right to divorcees, flagging clearly where it stood on the social issues of the day. In time, as divorce rates increased, this would cause no end of problems in individual parishes, and mark the Mothers' Union as an outdated institution.

In England, grounds for divorce other than adultery or "aggravated" adultery were a long time coming. In 1923, as we have noted, women could finally divorce their husbands on the grounds of simple adultery. In 1937, other grounds were also recognized, including wife-beating. Until the second half of the nineteenth century, wife-beating had not been punished in law — a circumstance based on the principle that a husband had the right to "moderate correction" of his wife. This principle, previously enshrined in canon law, was finally abolished in England in 1891. It is sobering to reflect on how very recent this about-face is in Western society, and to realize that the Church supported the right of "moderate correction" on the basis that, as the husband was legally responsible for his wife's actions, he had the right to control her.

It was the passing of the various Married Woman's Property Acts in the 1880s and 1890s that forced an end to this legal absurdity. Once married women could own property and have a legal entity of their own, the need for this "correction" passed. These changes in the status of women were a direct result of the campaigning of the women's movement, which had grown apace in the United States and Britain from the middle of the nineteenth century. It is worth remembering that the churches had, almost universally, opposed the granting of any rights to women throughout this period and beyond, arguing that the subordination of women was an immutable scriptural truth.[21]

Until the 1960s, divorce law changed by the addition of more and more grounds for divorce. By the 1960s, there was a growing recognition of the artificiality of many of these grounds, and particularly the difficulty of distinguishing between innocent and guilty parties. The result was that most Western societies completely changed their concept of divorce between the 1960s and mid-1980s. They moved away from grounds and fault to the concept of "no fault." Now, the usual requirement for divorce is evidence of irremedial breakdown in terms of a specific period of time of separation. This has "transferred to the spouses themselves the definition of acceptable marital behaviour and conditions."[22]

During these changes in the twentieth century, where have the churches been? Again, the question is most complex for the Anglican Church. The Roman Catholic Church has stuck firmly to its "no divorce, no remarriage" line, though in practice the possibility of an annulment has allowed some people to circumvent the otherwise inflexible rule. The Orthodox Church, which has a married priesthood, allows its lay members to be divorced up to three times. The nonconformist or free churches have generally been quite liberal and flexible. Many a divorced Anglican resorted to these churches in past decades for remarriage. The Anglican Church, however, across the world, was forced to reexamine its own hardline attitude as it faced the challenge of the rising divorce rate.

In the first half of the twentieth century, its attitude became even more hardline, if that were possible, certainly as far as its own role was concerned. The debate, at one level, was whether the church should seek to influence the state in its legislating for all citizens, or whether it should seek only to protect its own adherents. One important book, published in 1912, thundered that marriage was utterly indissoluble, except by death. It held that remarriage was merely a form of adultery. This book, *Marriage in Church and State*, was revised and republished in 1947, its hardline views intact. In 1958, another history of the Anglican Church's attitude to marriage and divorce upheld that church's most rigorous attitude. A. R. Winnett wrote that easier divorce meant more divorce, thus putting society at risk. He maintained, further, that in the face of demand for easier divorce, the Church must stand firm, or risk betraying its Lord's teaching and its own mission. It was unthinkable that the Church should not stand by the "almost universal" rule that no remarriage should take place with the Church's rites while the other partner was still living. To change its mind would be a "betrayal of the steadfastness and heroism of those men and women who through difficulties and suffering are remaining faithful to their marriage vows."[23]

Until 1948, Lambeth Conferences were still insisting that divorced people could not be remarried in church, even when they were the "innocent" party. But just a few short years later, the winds of change would overturn this long-held and fiercely defended situation. In 1966, an official report of the Church of England recommended the doctrine of breakdown of a marriage rather than the old principle of (one-sided) fault, thus paving the way for new English divorce laws.[24]

By 1971, a Commission on the Christian Doctrine of Marriage had recommended remarriage in church "with certain safeguards." In a generous report, this Commission noted that Christian congregations were "scandalised" neither by the presence of divorcees or remarried people in their midst nor by these people's participation in Holy Communion. There was, it said, a "moral consensus" within the Christian family that remarriage was morally acceptable.

The report went on to speak of grace: "An adequate doctrine of grace can loose as well as bind, forgive as well as bless, create again as well as create at first ... " It recognized that well-intentioned marriages break down, and that divorced people could enter into "new unions in good faith." Some of these unions showed "such evident features of stability, complementarity, fruitfulness and growth as to make them comparable with satisfactory first marriages."[25]

Not surprisingly, given its stringent constitution and highly diverse regional differences, the Australian Anglican Church struggled for decades to reach its current situation. In 1973, a

Commission set up by General Synod to report on the situation brought down a majority finding in favor of church remarriage for divorced people "with due safeguards." The two members who dissented argued that the "deprivation of the church service is part of the price which must be paid for past failure ... "

This minority opinion signalled the coming controversy. While a canon to allow remarriage of divorced persons was passed provisionally[26] by General Synod in 1973, its status was called into question by a reference to the Appellate Tribunal, the Australian Anglican Church's highest legal body. "Was the canon constitutional?" was the question asked of the Tribunal by some who were opposed to its passage. The following year, the Tribunal ruled it was unconstitutional, forcing the whole process to begin again.

Divorce law reform in Australia during the 1960s had led to the landmark *Family Law Act* of 1975, which abolished all other grounds of divorce bar separation for twelve months. Australia now had "no fault" divorce. The divorce rate rose rapidly so that by the late 1970s, the pressure on the Church from all sides was mounting. Bishops, clergy, and congregations were agitating for a more realistic and compassionate church response.

In 1979, in this climate, a second reference to the Tribunal saw the 1974 decision set aside. The majority ruled there was no constitutional bar to divorced persons' remarrying in the church in Australia. Against this background, a new canon was brought to General Synod in 1981, where once more it received provisional assent. In the dioceses, twenty-one of the twenty-four dioceses approved it, with the dioceses of Sydney, Ballarat, and Armidale dissenting. It is interesting to note that these are the dioceses most strongly opposed to the ordination of women to this day. They represent the extreme Evangelical wing of the church (Sydney and Armidale) and the extreme Anglo-Catholic wing (Ballarat). But the bill received the two-thirds majorities once again in General Synod in 1985, and the canon became church law. Sydney and Armidale have still refused to pass the canon.

The high rates of divorce in Western society in the wake of "no fault" divorce legislation show little sign of abating. In Australia today, about 40 per cent of marriages can expect to end in divorce. One hundred years ago, that figure was below 1 per cent, though about 10 per cent of marriages at that time ended in separation without formal divorce.[27] Do these figures prove that the doomsayers were right, that easy divorce means that too many marriages are entered into unwisely, and that family life and therefore the very structure of society has been dealt a mortal blow? Have modern church leaders simply capitulated to the pressures of secular society, when they should have upheld traditional standards, as has the Church of Rome?

Phillips has argued that the modern level of marriage breakdown is not caused by character weakness, moral slackness, irresponsibility or even the growth of secular society so much as the vastly different climate in which marriages now function. "The argument for marriage stability in the past," he has written, "rests ... not on assessments of the quality of conjugal relationships in earlier times, but on the broad social, economic and demographic contexts of marriage."[28] In other words, marriages in the past were not necessarily intrinsically any better than they are today; they held together because there was no other real choice. Today there are other options.

The churches cannot hold back this tide. The societal forces that propped up many intrinsically destructive marriage relationships have gone forever. Bad marriages in modern times will break down whatever the churches' attitude, because people no longer need to tolerate the intolerable. People will seek healing and renewal through subsequent marriages, with or without the Church. In Western society, the Anglican and Protestant churches – those churches most in tune with the realities of modern life – have changed their minds on the issue of divorce since the sixteenth century, the beginning of the modern era. They have been forced to confront not just the situation around them, but the ultimate implications of their whole theological understanding of sex and marriage.

As long as marriage – and its sexual component – was regarded as a union designed primarily for procreation, and not for companionship and holistic communion, then it inevitably had an almost mechanical basis. The notion of indissolubility could be maintained because the reality of the marriage was not deemed to be threatened by any problems the couple faced within their personal relationship. The problems were unfortunate, but peripheral. Once the "procreation" base was challenged, thereby giving way to an understanding of marriage as being a living relationship between two people, then the possibility of the death of the marriage had eventually to be faced.

The Protestant churches faced the implications of this developing theology far earlier than the Anglican Church, which clung to a proto-Roman position until the last couple of decades. Exactly why this was so deserves some further exploration, though the answer doubtless lies somewhere in the Anglican Church's unique "Catholic but reformed" status. Its persistent leanings toward Rome keep its reforming tendencies in constant check, as witnessed by its struggle with the question of the ordination of women.

Having made the shift, however, the Anglican Church is now, on the whole, comfortable with the new reality. Though numerous clergy once protested that their consciences would never allow them to remarry divorcees in church, very few actually hold to that position today. Most of them have come to understand that there is grace to free, to heal, to re-create, as the 1971 English report said, and that this grace can be acknowledged through the healing process of a church marriage. The Church is now increasingly comfortable with divorced and remarried clergy, and even with divorced and remarried bishops. The Australian Anglican Church currently has two remarried men in active episcopal orders. The Church of England, characteristically moving more slowly, has found greater difficulty in accepting remarried clergy. This suggests that that church still holds to the notion that the clergy represent a separate caste, a point to which we will return.

The Church of Rome, however, has made no concessions on the issue of divorce at all. It maintains an absolute bar on divorce, on the grounds that validly contracted marriages are dissoluble only by death. Only the availability of an annulment process, for marriages deemed not to have been validly contracted in the first place, has allowed some leeway for devout Catholics struggling with marital difficulties. This consistent rigidity could be interpreted as maintaining true teaching despite secular pressures. However, the agony this causes so many Catholics, whose second marriages are unrecognized and who are barred from the central sacrament of their faith because of it, suggests otherwise. As in so many other areas of morals for the Roman Catholic Church, there is no allowance at all for a development of doctrine.

Why not, when the other churches – despite a hard struggle – have conceded development? The answer is surely tied up with the question of priestly celibacy. By refusing to allow a married clergy, the Roman Catholic Church has turned its back on a full exploration of the nature of marriage and its holiness, and the inevitable implications that would proceed from that. It has also denied itself the life experience that married clergy would bring to these issues.

This is never more apparent than in its continuing total opposition to the use of artificial contraception, when other churches have accepted its use. But this still required a substantial change of mind for those other churches.

Given the preeminent Christian teaching that marriage was primarily, if not solely, for the purpose of procreation, it is not surprising that the Christian Church's original stance on contraception was one of total opposition. If marriage is for procreation, then to prevent this by any deliberate means other than abstinence (which was highly recommended for different reasons) was wrong. Over the centuries there have been nuances in the interpretation of this situation, but the central prohibition remained firmly in place till the twentieth century, bolstered by the Church's antipathy to sexual pleasure. Its persistent opposition to such pleasure even within marriage was a further deterrent to contraceptive practices. For with contraception, the effective brake placed on sexual pleasure by the threat of conception was eliminated. These two factors, and the continuing insistence that marital love was somehow divorced from sexual intimacy, prevented the Church from understanding that sex within marriage might have a role in deepening the total marital relationship. So the growing realization in the reformed churches that marriage primarily consisted in mutuality rather than procreation or remedy failed to influence their thinking about contraception until comparatively recently.[29]

Like divorce, the issue did not become a major one for any of the churches until artificial contraception was already being widely used. The development of the women's movement during the nineteenth century, combined with the advent of improved life expectancy, saw the beginnings of agitation for greater availability of contraceptive devices. Falling birth rates reveal that such devices were widely in use in Europe by the end of the nineteenth century. But the churches remained opposed, at least initially. However, because the numbers of women involved in the workforce increased as the twentieth century progressed, and because this was combined with a more positive attitude to sex and a developing concern with overpopulation and the risks that it posed for the planet, a dramatic sea-change finally occurred.

The change was ushered in tentatively, however, and hedged about with many qualifications. In 1930, the Lambeth Conference of Anglican Bishops gave cautious approval to the use of contraception by married couples where there was "a clearly-felt moral obligation to limit or avoid parenthood" and a "morally sound reason for avoiding complete abstinence." However, the conference recorded "its strong condemnation of the use of any methods of conception control from motives of selfishness, luxury or mere convenience." This was a limited reversal of the opposition expressed at two earlier conferences in 1908 and 1920. And it marked the first substantial approval given by any church to artificial contraception.

The subsequent resolution passed by the 1958 conference came from an entirely different thought-world:

> The Conference believes that the responsibility for deciding upon the number and frequency of children has been laid by God upon the consciences of parents everywhere: that this planning, in such ways as are mutually acceptable to husband and wife in Christian conscience, is a right and important factor in Christian family life and should be the result of positive choice before God. Such responsible parenthood, built on obedience to all the duties of marriage, requires a wise stewardship of the resources and abilities of the family as well as a thoughtful consideration of the varying population needs and problems of society and the claims of future generations.[30]

That it came a decade before the Church of Rome would prohibit artificial contraception in *Humanae Vitae* is surely telling. However, the Anglican church fathers were still uncomfortable with real sexual freedom in marriage. In Resolutions 112 and 113, they condemned "sins of self-indulgence and sensuality" in marriage, and commended "self-discipline and restraint." The ancient primacy of asceticism was still alive, if no longer as strong as it once had been.

The committee that had prepared these resolutions had produced a thoughtful report that examined carefully the arguments about the purposes of marriage. While it acknowledged the purpose of procreation, it gave equal weight to sexual union for relational reasons:

> Husbands and wives owe to each other and to the depth and stability of their families the duty to express, in sexual intercourse, the love which they bear and mean to bear to each other. Sexual intercourse is not by any means the only language of earthly love, but it is, in its full and right use, the most intimate and the most

revealing; it has the depth of communication signified by the Biblical word so often used for it, "knowledge"; it is a giving and receiving in the unity of two free spirits which is in itself good (within the marriage bond) and mediates good to those who share it. Therefore is is utterly wrong to urge that, unless children are specifically desired, sexual intercourse is of the nature of sin. It is also wrong to say that such intercourse ought not to be engaged in except with the willing intention to procreate children.[31]

This paragraph represents perhaps the most radical reversal in all the long centuries of Christian teaching on sexuality. It overturns not only the concept of procreation as primary cause, but also notions of marital sex as remedy for sin. At long last, it allows that sex is not only a valid expression of marital love, but actually the preeminent one. Though there is no hint of distaste for sex, there is as yet no acknowledgment of the sheer joy and pleasure of sex. It remains a "duty." But perhaps we should not be surprised. Pleasure and play have remained the most difficult concepts of all for theologians to embrace, whether in sexuality or anywhere else! The human capacity for fun is perhaps the last great challenge for a true theology of the human person.

This report has been described as marking a watershed in the Anglican approach to moral problems in that the concept of "moral consensus" as an instigator of theological revision was used to effect. An influential Bishop of Durham, Ian Ramsey, noted that "the status of the theology used in the argument was subordinate to the moral claim which in one way or another it was endeavouring to articulate." Reflecting on this comment, the writers of the 1971 Church of England report on divorce commented that "at times the Church may have moral insight prior to and at least as fundamental as the theological insight necessary to explain it." In 1958, the Lambeth Bishops had been "called upon to ratify a decision made in Christian consciences and acted upon for many years before." Was the divorce-and-remarriage debate another instance of moral consensus, "where the Church could be called upon to make provision for remarriage in the light of a moral judgement which has already formed itself, or is in the process of formation, within the Christian community ... ?"[32]

On the evidence, it seems clear that that is exactly what happened, on the issue both of contraception and of divorce. Christian communities, acting in good faith and on the basis of their own consciences, had decided that both contraception and remarriage after divorce were acceptable practices. In fact, by the time of the 1971 divorce report, the authors asked whether the moral consensus on divorce and remarriage had not moved to such a point that failure to allow divorcees to remarry in church was causing the greater offense.[33] Certainly by the time remarriage was formally allowed in Australian Anglican churches in the second half of the 1980s, the Anglican Church's record on the matter was a subject of deep offense and even scandal for many people. The Roman Catholic hierarchy's persistent refusal to countenance a more humane and realistic attitude to divorce and contraception remains a cause of offense and scandal among many in its own communities.

It is manifestly clear, from this brief survey, that mainstream Christian churches have changed their minds substantially on fundamental issues of Christian sexual theology and practice. It is also clear that theological exploration alone, or in isolation, has never been the primary motive. The churches have always seemed to require the urgent and persistent prodding of community need in order to initiate change. Sadly, the churches themselves have not been the major initiators. But, barring the Church of Rome, they have finally acted, often in complete reversal of earlier stances, when moral consensus has finally required it of them. Is moral consensus requiring yet more change in this area from the churches?

7

CHANGE IN
THE MODERN ERA ■

Moral consensus, rather than theological imperative, has clearly been the driving force behind the Church's radically altered stance on divorce and contraception in recent decades. And it is moral consensus that is now pushing Christian thinking toward a radical shift in its attitude to de facto and homosexual relationships, which have become the latest issues in sexual morality to challenge the status quo. There are signs that some cautious reevaluation is occurring in both these areas, and once again the Anglican Church offers the most interesting case study of this continuing process of change.

On both these issues, the evidence is that the Anglican Church is locked in a bitterly controversial struggle at the present time. While responsible, representative committees have begun tentatively to explore the boundaries of these areas, reactionary forces are ensuring that there will be no easy about-face. As in all the previous sexuality debates across the centuries, conservative church people are whipping up the paralyzing fear of the supposedly dire consequences of "opening the floodgates," and so rallying normally sensible and compassionate people to their side.

In the first chapter, we looked at the widespread acceptance of de facto relationships in modern Western society, an acceptance made possible by the effectiveness of modern forms of artificial contraception. This acceptance is also strong among regular churchgoers. It is even strong among clergy, who know full well that most of the couples they marry have been either living together for some period of time already or at least enjoying a full sexual relationship. But at an official level, the Church is loath to acknowledge this acceptance, and so such couples rarely feel able to worship regularly. If they feel unwelcome before marriage, it is highly unlikely that they will be disposed to regular church attendance after marriage.

The recent lectures on human sexuality given by Melbourne's Anglican Archbishop, Dr Keith Rayner, offer a reliable guide to the Church's official view at the present time. Without condemning all de facto relationships, and while demonstrating a real sympathy for some of the motivations behind them, Archbishop Rayner nevertheless declares that the Church "cannot endorse living together outside marriage as God's will."[1] This is in fact a harsh judgment, and one that ignores the long and valuable tradition of "betrothal" in Western society – a tradition that persisted well into the nineteenth century.

By contrast, the latest report from the Church of England, *Something to Celebrate: Valuing Families in Church and Society*, takes a more constructive approach. It points out, quite correctly, that "theologically and morally, what makes a marriage is the freely given consent and commitment in public of both partners to live together for life." The wedding ceremony solemnizes and blesses this consent entered into by the couple. Cohabitation, it argues, is often what may be called a "pre-ceremonial marriage." In the light of this, the report suggests that the Church needs to abandon the practise of calling cohabitation "living in sin." It states that this is a most unhelpful way of characterizing the lives of cohabitees:

> It has the effect of reducing cohabitation in all its complexity of intentions and variety of forms to a single, sensationalist category. Theologically and ethically it represents a serious failure to treat people as unique human beings. It perpetuates the widespread misconception that sex is sinful and that sin is only about sex.[2]

The report goes on to recommend that cohabitees be welcomed into congregational life. It warns that any serious evangelism in modern society must take the situation of cohabitees seriously, as the vast majority of people the Church is seeking to reach are living together.

Not surprisingly, the report immediately generated controversy. One member of the working party that fashioned the report resigned in protest as it reached its final stages. Dr Alan Storkey, a conservative Evangelical, is reported to have condemned the report because it "implicitly moves away from seeing marriage and the conjugal family as the universal pattern for human sexual relationships." That is precisely what the report did, but Dr Storkey perhaps failed to realize that the report was merely recognizing that marriage and the conjugal family had not been a "universal pattern," except for a brief period in very recent times. At both extremes of the Anglican churchmanship scale – both of them conservative bastions – came more damning condemnation. The English press reported Ecclesia, an Anglo-Catholic group, as saying that the report deserved "absolute and outright condemnation." An Evangelical leader said it was "riddled with the discredited permissive thinking of the 1960s." The report "attempts to be more welcoming to sinners than Jesus Christ," said Mr Philip Gore in a statement that was presumably not intended to be a compliment. Yet another detractor saw the report as a Trojan horse for a much greater liberalization yet to come.

Such controversy was not unexpected. Every time sexual morality issues are raised publicly in the Church, condemnation of anything that hints at a more liberal approach is certain to follow. When such issues are actually debated in synods, the result is a foregone conclusion. As with the sexuality debate in Melbourne Synod in 1993, referred to in Chapter 1, it is hard for the advocates of a moral liberal view to win the day. The rhetoric of certainty, of Gospel values, of holding the line against those dreaded floodgates, is usually extremely persuasive. Even people who would privately take a more liberal stance feel compelled to support publicly what is presented as the Church's "traditional" position. Experience shows that capitulation comes only when the battle has already been well and truly won outside the Church, over a period of decades, as in the case of changes to the Church's attitude to divorce and contraception.

Though most of the mainstream churches have accepted the practice of contraception, they have so far failed to understand its implications for human relationships. Officially, most would still wish to confine contraceptive practice to within marriage, though most would also acknowledge its value in preventing unwanted pregnancies – and therefore unnecessary abortions – outside marriage. But the fundamental change in male–female relationships that safe and reliable forms of contraception have provided remains unexplored. So far the churches have failed to understand its significance for their "no sex outside marriage" rule, a rule that may well have had more to do with the protection of women and property in a pre-contraceptive age than with intrinsic values.

More problematic is the Church's response to homosexual unions. This is another area in which the moral consensus of the wider community and among churchgoers is increasingly pushing the Church to reevaluate its position. While this book is not the place to attempt a historical survey of the Church's condemnation of homosexuality, it is nevertheless concerned with the implications for this area that can be drawn from its changing views on heterosexuality.

On the basis of a few isolated verses of Scripture, the Church has built a teaching that, almost universally, has condemned homosexual practices as at least immoral and at worst a perversion and abomination. No distinction has been made in the tradition between monogamous, loving same-sex relationships and homosexual activity that is exploitative, abusive or promiscuous. Even homosexual orientation has been presented as sinful in some interpretations of church law.

In the contemporary Church, few would still condemn homosexual orientation *per se*, and few – within the mainstream churches at least – would describe AIDS as the wrath of God for homosexual activity. But beyond that, there is considerable disagreement. Just within Australian Anglicanism, responses range from the measured, realistic, and compassionate assessment made by the late John Gaden to the narrow, judgmental document currently in circulation among Melbourne Evangelicals.[3]

Theologians such as John Gaden have been concerned to demonstrate the inadequacy of condemning all homosexual activity on the basis of the limited scriptural evidence. He and others have also argued that the biblical authors, in this area as well as in the area of the role of women, were hampered by a faulty understanding of human biology and sexuality. The Church's long struggle to come to terms with biblical imperatives and the reality of the dynamics of heterosexuality, as we have seen, should alert us to the extent of the problems it must face in dealing with homosexuality. It is simply not good enough to quote isolated verses and insist that this is what "the Bible says." Isolated verses that condemned a public ministry for women, such as 1 Timothy 2:11–15, continue to be used to argue that women should neither preach nor have any spiritual authority.[4]

Once again, the wider community has come to terms with the issue of homosexuality much more readily than have the churches. Homosexuality has been decriminalized in most parts of the Western world, though not yet in the Australian island state of Tasmania. Homosexual culture and lifestyle has become open to the wider public through large-scale public events such as the Sydney Gay and Lesbian Mardi Gras. Antidiscrimination laws have ensured that homosexual partnerships can claim many of the privileges of heterosexual de facto relationships, and such partnerships are increasingly open. Parenting issues remain the last major concern in the general community.

For the Church, however, it would be fair to say the situation is one of stalemate. Despite all the generosity of approach from Gaden and others, the Church remains frozen because it has tied itself up in the "no sex outside marriage" rule. That rule, so simple, so straightforward, answers all the criteria for those who want the overriding requirement of certainty and clear teaching on moral issues. If life were straightforward and human relationships and needs were completely unambiguous, it might well be a satisfactory rule. But patently it does not meet the real needs of flesh-and-blood women and men seeking honest and realistic guidelines. Rarely, indeed, has it ever met these needs. Like other rules once highly esteemed but now, in most mainstream churches, abandoned – rules such as "marriage is totally indissoluble" and "priests must be celibate" – it does not give life. Certainly it cannot give life to those for whom, because of their homosexual orientation, it offers no hope of relationship, ever.

So why do the churches persist with it in the face of so much evidence that even devout churchgoers no longer expect blind obedience to the letter of the rule? Certainly one reason must be the long struggle of the Church to control human sexuality. In its earliest centuries, the Church imposed that control through the myriad regulations that it devised in order to limit even marital sexual activity, including its prohibition on artificial contraception. This developed into even stricter control over the lives of clergy, followed by the increasing imposition of the celibacy law.

By the medieval period, the Church was moving to bring marriage itself under its sway, as it developed an elaborate doctrine of the sacramental nature of marriage – a comparatively late innovation. Its iron grip on this area prevented the advent of divorce until the demographic changes of the modern period made this no longer a realistic option. Similarly the women's movement, and safe and reliable forms of contraception, have combined to overthrow the need for absolute control by either Church or State over sex and marriage.

But the churches have invested so much of their energy over the centuries in this area of control that to lose it entirely could threaten their very identity. For centuries, the Christian Church has functioned as the moral policeman for the State, ensuring that people conformed to the requirements of their particular society. It upheld the status quo, encouraging submission to God, king, and country, to the feudal lord and the local squire. It sacralized classism, the notion of "each man in his station," and romanticized notions of meek and mild children, and pure and lowly womanhood. In latter years, under the onslaught of democratic principles, that influence has shrunk to the entirely domestic sphere. The exaltation of the nuclear family, abiding by "traditional" expectations, has become almost the central tenet of some church communities. Without it, there is not much left.

This question of identity is probably a stronger reason for resistance to change in this area than many realize. One of the Church's persistent sins is its tendency to see itself, or its clergy, as a separate caste, and therefore holier than anyone else. The fourth-century synod of Elvira that sparked clerical celibacy by introducing special rules for married clergy was almost certainly motivated by a desire to establish the clergy as a caste of specially holy people. The local church's regulations on marital sexuality were already stringent enough to ensure that its members were clearly "set apart" from their non-Christian neighbors; the demand for continent marriage among the clergy elevated them to yet another plane.

So the growing demand for a totally celibate priesthood ensured that the clergy were of an order different to that of the laity. Even in modern Western societies, Catholic clergy retain a mystique – manifested in the laity's grudging obedience – that married Protestant clergy have long since lost. It was at least one of the aims of the reformers that clergy should be restored to a position of effective leadership of the laity. However, permission to marry did not obliterate this ancient temptation to caste status in Protestant clergy, as we will see.

And the temptation is not confined to the clergy. In recent sexuality debates in the churches, it is not hard to discern the desire to impose strict guidelines on Christians for the purpose of marking them out as "different." The rules become a badge that is actually worn with pride. Christians of a fundamentalist persuasion, be they evangelical or from some other conservative position, revel in the notion that they are manifestly "counter-cultural." The logic is disarmingly simple. The Church should be counter-cultural; adopting rules on sex and marriage that are stricter than anyone else's is obviously counter-cultural, and clearly seen as such. *Ergo*, it must be right to insist on such rules.

It is not, of course, only in the sexuality area that exclusionary tactics are used to protect Christian identity. The modern debate on baptism and Christian initiation is a clear example of this process still at work. It is also another manifestation of the desire for control, for differentiation. This is not the place to pursue such an issue, except to say in passing that the Church always seems to lose the plot when it succumbs to the seductive temptation to exclude, no matter what the grounds. It ceases to be the community of the Incarnate One, and becomes instead a sect of the legalists.

Perhaps the Church also clings to these last vestiges of its past control because the option to change is so very demanding. As any participant in a debate on sexuality in the churches can testify, it is very hard work to change minds in this area. Church communities who have staked their identity on rules of personal conduct reject any attempt to overthrow these rules. Some people are threatened by the challenge to a morality that has become for them a shield against the dangerous exploration of their own real selves. Others, while perfectly willing to confront their own situation honestly, find it easier to support a new "double standard" than to challenge it openly. They know full well how ugly the sexuality debate can be in the synods, councils and commissions of the church as vested interests resist so profound a change.

A "double standard" – both old-style and new – is at work in many of the churches today. The older version survives in the Roman Catholic Church. The papal rules against clerical marriage and sexual activity remain as stringent as ever, except – surprisingly – for married Anglican clergy who have "gone to

Rome," principally in protest at the ordination of women. But though Catholic clergy are forbidden to marry, many in Australia today have semipermanent quasi-marital relationships, kept hidden from their superiors and their parishioners.

In the Anglican and Protestant churches, the new "double standard" means that modern community standards are now generally acceptable, and even cautiously given approval, but not for the clergy. We have seen that the recent English General Synod report recommended a much higher level of acceptance of de facto relationships. It even recommended acceptance of them within the Christian community: "Congregations should welcome cohabitees, listen to them, learn from them and co-operate with them so that all may discover God's presence in their lives and in our own … "[5]

The same report recommended that gay and lesbian families should "find a ready welcome within the whole family of God." This was in line with the more cautious welcome extended by the earlier influential report by the Church of England's House of Bishops, *Issues in Human Sexuality*. That statement, while not able to commend same-sex partnerships, called on congregations to welcome such couples as members. The language is supremely cautious, but nevertheless surprisingly generous.[6]

The bishops, however, reveal that they are still captive to an outdated understanding of human sexuality. Heterosexual activity serves "the purposes of procreation," they write:

> Furthermore, since it is the interaction of the male and female genital organs which makes procreation possible, that too must be part of God's purpose … In short, the biological evidence is at least compatible with a theological view that heterosexual physical union is divinely intended to be the norm.[7]

Heterosexual unions, in every way, reflect "their essential place in God's providential order." They are, therefore, truly "natural" in a way that homosexual unions never can be.

Though the rhetoric is careful and gracious, the underlying message is clear: homosexual unions are not as fully "natural" as heterosexual ones, because they do not fully reflect the clear divine will of the Creator that is expressed in the capacity for procreation.

How sad that the bishops seem to have reverted to the Church's earlier view – what might be called a "pre-contraceptive" view. In the ground-breaking report "The Family in Contemporary Society," which enabled the 1958 Lambeth Conference of Bishops to pioneer the acceptance of artificial contraception, the role of sexual function for reasons of companionship and support was given equal status with the procreative purpose, as we have seen. "It was not good for man to be alone, and God made a helpmeet for him," the report reminds its readers. In this context, it is of course talking of woman as the helpmeet for man, but it stresses, in a radical revision of the Church's ancient teachings, that "relationship" is "rooted in God's creative purpose equally with the procreative function of sexuality." Sexual activity within a committed relationship is just as important for relational reasons as it is for reproductive reasons. If this truly means what it says, then the corollary is that sexual activity does not have to be even potentially procreative to be "natural," and capable of carrying the divine purposes of God.

The 1958 report opened the door to a fresh understanding of homosexual union as also being "divine," if it answered the Genesis precept that it is not good for man to be alone. But since then, few theologians have dared to go through that door, preferring to condemn many men (and women) to a life alone, even though the biblical teaching is clear that this is not "good." The suffering and loneliness the Church has forced so many gay people to endure demonstrates forcibly this Genesis truth.

Despite the 1958 report, the bishops in 1991 revealed that they were still wedded to the belief that only heterosexual unions were truly "natural." Even the best faithful monogamous same-sex unions were not as "faithful a reflection of God's purposes in creation as the heterophile," they said, and so they were not able to accept same-sex partnerships among the clergy. The bishops state that the Church's traditional stance of requiring clergy to "live the Gospel," to be moral exemplars for the people, means that "certain possibilities are not open to the clergy by comparison with the laity, something that in principle has always been accepted."[8] As in fourth-century Spain, when the growing ideal of asceticism saw even married clergy required to be totally continent – and therein "living the Gospel" – so homosexual clergy today are required to live a life of total sexual abstinence in order to demonstrate the modern highest ideal: that only heterosexual sexual activity is truly "of God." In the same way, divorce and remarriage has been so much more problematic for clergy than for laity, particularly in the Church of England, though the Australian Anglican Church's ready acceptance of the same standard for both clergy and laity does not seem to have caused any "moral exemplar" problems.

The reality is, of course, that the Anglican Church, like the Catholic Church, has a significant proportion of gay clergy. Like heterosexual clergy in the Catholic Church, some of the Anglican gay clergy live in long-term partnerships with other men or women. The exact nature of these relationships is kept carefully hidden, however, as the current church leadership in most Australian dioceses would not be prepared to turn a blind eye, let alone accept them openly. Even in the Episcopal Church of the United States – one of the more liberal branches of the Anglican Communion – progressive bishops who have attempted to ordain openly gay clergy in recent times have faced legal challenges mounted by conservatives.

Potential ordinands who admit to homosexual relationships are generally refused ordination, placing gay people who believe they have a vocation to the priesthood in a real dilemma. Some believe they have no alternative but to keep silent about their lifestyle, and so live with a sense of unworthy compromise; others sadly forgo what they believe is God's calling. The Church is often the loser, as it has lost some people of great gifts and deep integrity. Many perceptive churchgoers can testify to the great gifts homosexual clergy offer the Church, in terms of a high capacity for pastoral care born of their own experience of pain and rejection, a sensitivity to the needs of those who do not fit the conventional patterns of family life, and artistic flair.

The alternatives for gay clergy at present are limited. Either they remain celibate, if they can, and despite the fact that it might be a difficult and life-denying choice for them personally; they maintain a full relationship in absolute secrecy, with all the burdens that that entails; or they indulge in occasional promiscuous episodes. These are in fact the same limited options open to Catholic heterosexual clergy. That the deepest human needs of all these clergy should be forcibly denied, for the sake of offering society an entirely unrealistic and unhelpful "moral exemplar," is painful not just for them, but for their many friends within the Church. It also forces many of them to live a "double life," with all the pain and hypocrisy that that entails.

The parallels with the situation facing the sixteenth-century reformers are interesting. The fact that supposedly celibate clergy were often sexually active was bringing the Church into disrepute. Most people revile hypocrisy as a far more serious sin than simple failure to live up to an impossible ideal. The reformers believed the Church's attempts to provide real moral guidance for people in a rapidly changing world was compromised by enforced celibacy. As we have seen, they were in no doubt that celibacy was the ideal for the clergy, and provided the moral example *par excellence*, for sexual abstinence was then the highest ideal for all Christians. But the ideal was hardly realistic for the vast bulk of the laity, in a society that was founded on the interlocking networks of the family. They needed a moral example that taught an acceptable pattern of sexual activity, and the reformers came to the conclusion that a married clergy could provide this, even if it amounted to compromising the traditionally highest ideal of chastity in the clergy. In time, of course, it created a totally reverse "highest ideal."

So clergy were free to marry, to provide a model of marriage and family life to their contemporaries. It was the lesser of two evils, but it offered a realistic and manageable model for lay people to emulate. In the last decade of the twentieth century, the Church needs to accept that it may have to offer a realistic model for homosexuals as well as for heterosexuals even if, for some church leaders, this also involves a "lesser of two evils" approach. Over the last twenty years, homosexual culture and lifestyle have become widely accepted in Western society. Younger people in particular are comfortable with a world that includes openly gay people and gay relationships. When the English bishops argued that "a significant number of people at this time" would find it difficult to accept openly gay people as "messengers, watchmen and stewards of the Lord," thus limiting their capacity to offer pastoral ministry, they were revealing their captivity to the views of the older generation to which they themselves belong.[9]

It goes without saying that, even in the more liberal climate of contemporary society, gay people still face greater pressures than straight people. Like the divorcees of a generation ago, they can still be stigmatized as failures, people who do not live up to the highest ideals of their society. From the sixteenth century onwards, married clergy offered society a model of acceptable sexuality and sanctified domesticity, creating a revolution in standards that even the Church of Rome itself adopted in time, though only for its laity.

Much more recently, divorced and remarried clergy have helped to provide a compassionate realization that second marriages can be a source of grace and new beginnings for people scarred by earlier hurt and failure. This does not for one moment detract from the Church's "ideal" standard of the permanence of marriage. If anything, it gives it greater recognition, and reinforces the notion that it is the content and not the form of marriage that is ultimately important.

Before the Reformation, clergy who could not remain celibate knew that if they were in a monogamous relationship they were just as sinful, in the eyes of the Church, as if they were wildly promiscuous. For some, this doubtless made promiscuity the more attractive option, as it carried no responsibility. Gay people are in much the same situation in the eyes of the Church today, despite the English bishops' cautious acceptance of gay couples as members of the congregation. That "welcome" is still so grudging, so discreet, that it offers little to gays in the wider community. The Church offers them no model of monogamy at all to attract them from the life-denying captivity of promiscuity into which the dynamics of rejection can so easily force them. The Church offers no understanding of their need for love and acceptance within an open relationship of trust and commitment.

If gay clergy were permitted to live in open monogamous relationships committed to the best standards sought by partners in heterosexual marriage, the gift to the Church as a whole as well as to the wider community would be incalculable. It would release not only the considerable gifts of many talented individuals in the ordained ministry: it would signal a whole new level of trust in, and an openness toward, the reality of the human sex drive. Moreover, it would herald the dawning of a new respect for what it means to be fully human and fully alive, and facilitate recognition of the complexity and ambiguity of human nature. It would signify that human nature is not simple, and that a theology of the human person cannot be simplistic. It would offer to the wider community realistic models of relationship that bring life and grace. In a time when the Church rightly condemns Western society's obsession with the pursuit of sexual pleasure as an end in itself, and the fruitless search for perfect romantic happiness,[10] it would offer real alternatives for the full range of human need.

If the Church were to move down this path – and if it is to avoid cutting itself off entirely from modern life it will have to do this sooner or later – then it would need to be careful that it did not set up these new "moral exemplars" in such a way that they became potentially destructive. The Australian Anglican General Synod Social Responsibilities Commission's report on the breakdown of clerical marriages identified pressure to model the perfect family as being a significant factor in clergy marriage breakdown. Specifically, it recommended a reexamination of the contemporary ordination vow, that the priest's family would offer "good examples to the flock of Christ."[11] This vow, introduced into the first reformed Ordinal of the Church of England in 1550, demonstrated clearly one of the reasons why the reformers insisted on clerical marriage. It may also have had a polemical purpose at the time, ensuring that it was abundantly clear that clerical marriage was now an established expectation. But in its present form in modern society, it has become a burden.

The long-term implications for the personal life of the priest and his family could not, of course, have been guessed at by the original framers of the ordination vow. But, in time, it would place an almost impossible demand on clergy families. The report on clergy marriage breakdown called for the omission of these references, or at least for the "rewording [of] them so that they reflect less the need to model a perfect family and more the need to engage positively in the care of significant human relationships." The new vow contained in *A Prayer Book for Australia* has in fact changed the promise significantly. Clergy will no longer promise that they and their families "will be good examples to the flock of Christ"; instead, they will strive to shape their lives and the life of their household, "according to the way of Christ." The "modelling" aspect has been eliminated.[12] This removes entirely the pressure to offer a model of perfection, substituting the more creative and realistic aim of working towards an ideal rather than embodying it.

In any case, expecting the clergy to offer a model of perfection, in any area of life, that the laity are not actually required to reach reinforces the notion that the clergy belong to a different caste. This is almost always counterproductive, because it is so alienating. The better model is surely that offered by the central Christian doctrine of Incarnation. Clergy – and laity – striving to live the way of Christ in the fulness of their humanity with all its struggles, mistakes, and moments of glory, offer the world a vision akin to that offered by Christ himself. There is a world of difference between this incarnational model and that of the cardboard-cutout, "dead-from-the-neck-down," music-hall parody of the parson, which rightly attracts the world's derision. The bloodless parson of the parody turns many people in need away from the Church, for fear of rejection and humiliation.

Does this mean anything goes? That the Church should mindlessly endorse any and all sexual behavior? Certainly not. It could be argued that the Church's long history of condemnation of the human sex drive and all sexual experience, which influenced the development of Western society so powerfully, is responsible for the recent "breakout" of sex in that society. The "anything goes" mentality and the obsession with sex themes – and particularly violent and abusive sex themes – in modern entertainment and culture are a backlash against the centuries of unhealthy sexual suppression and anti-women attitudes. Truly healthy cultural attitudes to sexuality need to be created, and the Church should be the leader in that drive.

But in order to do so, the Church will have to abandon its own obsession with simple certainties and simplistic rules. It will have to abandon the long shadows of asceticism that have been so life-denying. Instead, it will have to acknowledge the full diversity of human need and experience, abandon the pursuit of hard-and-fast rules, and help modern people formulate guidelines that encourage the best that is human in all relationships. As the feminist writer Janet Nelson pointed out in the Melbourne Synod debate on sex, there is a biblical measure most appropriate for this area, and that is, "by their fruits you shall know them":

> If we use this measure we could condemn as un-
> Christian what is destructive, degrading, exploitative
> and abusive in any sexual relationships, and we could

affirm as good those relationships which are marked by joy, peace, generosity, tenderness, compassion, mutual trust and love … [13]

CONCLUSION:
IF ONLY ...

■

Genesis, the first book of the Bible, has two accounts of Creation. In the first, men and women are created together, both in God's image, and are commanded to be fruitful and multiply (Genesis 1:26–28). In the second, the man is created first. God recognizes the loneliness of the solitary human. "It is not good that the man should be alone," God says, and so creates a female partner for the man out of the man's own flesh. "Therefore a man leaves his father and his mother and clings to his wife, and they become one flesh" (Genesis 2:18–24).

To feminist Christians – for obvious reasons – the first account of mutual creation is the more acceptable. The second account suggests female inferiority. Yet the Fathers of the Church, to a man, while insisting that women were a secondary creation, nevertheless based their theology of marriage on the first account. For in the first, the only reason for the coupling of man and woman is to be fruitful and multiply, and that formed the basis of the Fathers' entire understanding of the purpose of marriage. They declared that procreation was the first, indeed almost the sole, reason for marriage and therefore for sex in marriage, and so they built on procreation the whole edifice of traditional marriage theology. The demands of procreation required a mechanistic view of marriage, and with it, a theology of exclusivity, indissolubility, and a total prohibition on contraception.

It is not difficult to see why the Fathers and their successors should have preferred this version of the reason for marriage. In their exaltation of asceticism, and their consequent denial of sexual desire and attraction, the continuation of the human race was the only permissible reason for the sex act. Because of the physical limitations governing the number of children that any couple could desire or even create, a limitation was placed on sexual activity. It was a minimalist approach to sex and marriage – the approach of male celibates who preferred that all men should be as they were.

Certainly, they could not have based their theology of marriage and human relationships on the second account of Creation while upholding their preference for celibacy. "It is not good that the man should be alone" offers an entirely different rationale for marriage. It suggests that celibacy, or singleness in any form, is not the ideal for human beings at all, but rather that companionship, in every aspect of life, is God's vision. So companionship – in the one flesh of full sexual union – not procreation is the prime cause for marriage. This, not the demand of procreation, is why men and women create a new household, in which they "cling" to each other.

Had this "demand" of companionship been accepted by the Fathers as the basis of their theology of sex, marriage, and human relationships in general, it would have created a vastly different theology. It would not have allowed a mechanistic, legalistic view at all, but rather a realistic and compassionate model that promoted the relational needs of men and women above all else. In this model, there would have been no problem with contraception – as the relational need for sexual intimacy would have been paramount – and no rigid barrier to divorce. "No sex outside marriage" would have been harder to justify, particularly for those of homosexual orientation for whom conventional marriage was not an option. If it is not good for people to be alone, then it is not good for people to be attracted to those of the same sex. Sexual abstinence and celibacy would have been the exceptions, not the ideal, throughout Christian history. How different that history would have been!

And if only the same Fathers had taken the pastoral epistles as their biblical yardstick for the lifestyle of the clergy. In 1 Timothy 3:2 and Titus 1:6, clergy were expected to be married men. In fact, these are the least ambiguous and most direct biblical verses on clergy behavior overall, yet they were consistently overlooked in favor of far more ambiguous teachings on sexual abstinence, such as 1 Corinthians 7. Again, in an age wedded to the dualistic doctrines of sexual abstinence inherited from the Greco-Roman thought-world, the notion of priests as married men was abhorrent and therefore unthinkable – despite its biblical warrant. Even the reformers rarely cited the pastoral epistles in their impassioned pleas for clerical marriage, because they were still heirs to ascetical models of human excellence.

In the modern world, it is time that this unequivocal biblical basis for a fresh understanding of human relationships, based on nothing less than the holiness of sexual intimacy, was implemented urgently by all the churches.

The Roman Catholic Church has the longest journey to take in this area. Without a married priesthood or women priests, it will be extremely difficult for it to come to terms with the grave pastoral problems it faces because of its rules on contraception, marriage, and divorce. Only a married priesthood will help it overcome, in the long term, the scandal of priestly sexual abuse it is currently facing. Ugly as this scandal has been, it should at least have alerted church leaders to the extreme dangers of forcing all clergy into the pressure cooker of compulsory celibacy. A married clergy would not eliminate the problem of abuse entirely, any more than it has in the other churches, but it would at least control its proportions along with the level of hypocrisy they signal.

As so many of its adherents around the world would insist, the Roman Catholic Church must very soon confront the reality of the innate goodness of human sexuality, which must underpin change in this area. A rhetoric of the goodness of sex and marriage is totally unconvincing until it permits clergy to marry; a rhetoric of the equality of women is likewise unconvincing until women can be ordained.

Almost certainly because they have allowed their clergy to marry, the other churches have had to come to terms with the reality of human sexuality. But as the record shows, they came to terms with it not because of theological imperatives but because society's overwhelming needs drove them – sometimes kicking and screaming! – to the point of recognition. Often it was the moral consensus arrived at by the laity themselves that drove church leaders to change their minds. Married church leaders were at least sufficiently in touch with society to recognize this lay moral consensus, even if it was a belated recognition. While the Church may purport to "lead" the community in the area of personal morality, the reality is that it has been the community that has led the Church. Certainly the community has generally proved to be more realistic and more compassionate than those they might have expected to pastor them.

The Christian Church, over its 2000 years of history, has changed its mind often on issues of sex and marriage. There are no "certainties"; there are no tablets of stone. It is time that that was recognized, and the Church was freed to offer Christ's promise of life, in all its fullness, to all people.

GLOSSARY

anathema: enforced complete separation from the Church in every respect.

asceticism: self-denial through rigorous austerities, designed to purify the soul of all passions, particularly those of a sexual and bodily nature.

banns: the formal announcement, during divine service, of a forthcoming marriage. The practice, which is still observed in the Church of England, was designed to prevent unsuitable or bigamous marriages.

canon law: church law.

compline: the traditional name for the final daily service of prayer.

Convocation: the name given to the meetings of the clergy of the two Church of England provinces of Canterbury and York. Bishops, deans, archdeacons, and representative "lower" clergy meet under the chairmanship of their respective Archbishop.

ecclesiology: the study of the nature and structure of the Christian Church.

injunction: the name given to each of a series of Tudor royal proclamations on church affairs.

martyr: one who gives up their life because they refuse to deny their Christian faith while suffering persecution for it.

Mishnah: authoritative collection of Jewish oral law.

monastic movement: had its beginnings in the third century in Egypt, before spreading to the West in the fourth century. Monasteries allowed men and women to attempt to live lives of spiritual perfection away from the distractions of worldly life, under the discipline of vows of poverty, chastity, and obedience to the superior of the monastery or religious order. The commitment to chastity led, in some cases, to extreme manifestations of asceticism (see separate entry).

mortal sin: a grave sin that must be confessed before the taking of the sacraments. If unrepented, it is believed to lead to eternal damnation.

Pelagianism: theological teaching concerned with grace and free will, holding that human beings are endowed with a capacity to perform good works and accordingly are not in need of a special grace for the achievement of that end. The teaching takes its name from the fourth-century British monk Pelagius, who first formulated it.

recusant: a term used during the late-sixteenth century and into the seventeenth century in England for those who, retaining their allegiance to the Church of Rome, refused to attend the services of the established Church of England, as required by law for all English citizens.

synod: originally a meeting of the clergy and bishop of a diocese (the unit of church government, usually based on a geographic area); in modern times, a meeting of the bishop, clergy and representative lay people of a diocese.

transubstantiation: the belief that the whole substance of the bread and wine of the Holy Communion becomes the whole substance of the actual Body and Blood of Christ, though retaining the appearance of bread and wine. This belief was central to Roman Catholic eucharistic theology at the time of the Reformation; adherence to it thus became the mark of a true Catholic, while dissent from it became the mark of the Protestant.

venial sin: a sin of less gravity than a mortal sin (see separate entry), the confession of which is not held to be necessary for the taking of the sacraments.

APPENDIX
1 CORINTHIANS 7

Following are selected verses from 1 Corinthians 7, according to the Geneva Bible of 1560. Note that spelling has been modernized.

1 Now concerning the things whereof ye wrote unto me, It were good for a man not to touch a woman.

2 Nevertheless, to avoid fornication, let every man have his wife, and let every woman have her own husband.

3 Let the husband give unto the wife due benevolence, and likewise also the wife unto the husband.

4 The wife hath not the power of her own body, but the husband: and likewise also the husband hath not the power of his own body, but the wife.

5 Defraud not one another, except it be with consent for a time, that ye may give yourselves to fasting and prayer, and again come together that Satan tempt you not for your incontinency.

6 But I speak this by permission, not by commandment.

7 For I would that all men were even as I myself am: but every man hath his proper gift of God, one after this manner, and another after that.

8 Therefore I say unto the unmarried, and unto the widows, it is good for them if they abide even as I do.

9 But if they cannot abstain, let them marry: for it is better to marry than to burn.

10 And unto the married I command, not I, but the Lord, let not the wife depart from her husband.

11 But if she depart, let her remain unmarried, or be reconciled unto her husband, and let not the husband put away his wife ...

25 Now concerning virgins, I have no commandment of the Lord: but I give mine advice, as one that hath obtained mercy of the Lord to be faithful.

26 I suppose then this to be good for the present necessity: I mean that it is good for a man so to be.

27 Art thou bound unto a wife? Seek not to be loosed: art thou loosed from a wife? Seek not a wife.

28 But if thou takest a wife, thou sinnest not: and if a virgin marry, she sinneth not: nevertheless, such shall have trouble in the flesh: but I spare you ...

32 And I would have you without care. The unmarried careth for the things of the Lord, how he may please the Lord.

33 But he that is married, careth for the things of the world, how he may please his wife.

ENDNOTES ∎

CHAPTER 1

1 The debate is reported in the November 1993 edition of *SEE* (now *The Melbourne Anglican*), the monthly journal of the Melbourne Anglican Diocese.

2 A recent, authoritative exposition of the "traditional" Christian teaching on sexual morality can be found in *Human Sexuality: A Christian Perspective*, a series of four addresses delivered in St Paul's Cathedral, Melbourne, in October and November 1994 by Dr Keith Rayner, Archbishop of Melbourne, and published in booklet form by the Anglican Diocese of Melbourne. See also a contemporary restatement of the conservative Christian response to homosexuality in Peter Corney, *Homosexuality: A Christian Response*, EFAC Victoria (no date).

3 L. P. Hartley, *The Go-Between*, Penguin Books, Harmondsworth, 1958, p. 7.

4 The debate was the subject of my thesis, "The Defence of the Marriage of Priests in the English Reformation," for which a Ph.D. was awarded by the University of Melbourne in 1988. The other main research in this area is Eric Josef Carlson, "Clerical Marriage and the English Reformation," *Journal of British Studies*, 31, January 1992, pp. 1–31. Prof. Carlson's work, however, does not examine the theological or ecclesiological reasons for the change in the marital status of the clergy. An earlier examination of the literature is found in John K. Yost, "The Reformation Defense of Clerical Marriage in the Reigns of Henry VIII and Edward VI," *Church History*, 50, 1981, pp. 152–165. This is a brief discussion of the literature written in Tudor England up to 1553, combined with an attempt to discern evidence of specifically humanist thought within it. The clerical marriage debate is mentioned only in passing in the

more general works on the growth of the clerical profession in England, such as Rosemary O'Day, *The English Clergy: The Emergence and Consolidation of a Profession 1558–1642*, Leicester University Press, Leicester, 1979, or even in works looking at aspects of clerical married life, for example, Anne L. Barstow, "The First Generations of Anglican Clergy Wives: Heroines or Whores?", *Historical Magazine of the Protestant Episcopal Church*, 52, 1983, pp. 3–16.

5 3 James I cc. 25, 26, *Statutes of the Realm*, vol. IV, part II, London 1819, reprinted 1963.

6 Tricia Blombery and Philip Hughes, *Australian Families: Practices and Attitudes*, Christian Research Association Research Paper no. 1, June 1994, pp. 15–16.

7 *Ibid.*, p.7.

8 David Jenkins, the former controversial Bishop of Durham, England, has said that it is "rubbish" for the Church to try to offer "certainty" (in any area) because "(a) you can't; (b) they know it; and (c) you're cheating!" Quoted in "Can't Keep a Good God Down," *Melbourne Anglican*, March, 1995, p. 16.

9 Blombery and Hughes, *op. cit.*, pp. 10–15.

10 John R. Gillis, *For Better, for Worse: British Marriages, 1600 to the Present*, Oxford University Press, Oxford, 1985, p. 277. Though Gillis' study is confined to Britain, it is nevertheless applicable to Australia and other Western cultures.

11 *Ibid.*, p. 294.

12 *Ibid.*, pp. 12, 11.

13 Martin Ingram, *Church Courts, Sex and Marriage in England 1570–1640*, Cambridge University Press, Cambridge, 1987, pp. 131–132. In Europe, marriage law had been rationalized in 1563 by the Council of Trent to require public marriage before a priest in order that a marriage be valid, but in England, despite attempts at reform, the marriage law fixed by canon law in the twelfth century remained unaltered until the *Hardwicke Marriage Act* of 1753.

14 *Ibid.*, pp. 154–155. Most moralists at the time recognized these liaisons as being ambiguous; the sexual relationship within them

was generally not regarded to be as wrongful as other forms of extramarital sexual activity. Some, however, such as William Harrington, writing in 1528 (at the height of reform fervor) regarded sex within the betrothal period as "deadly sin."

15 *Ibid.*, p. 157. Ingram quotes as his sources Philip E. Hair, "Bridal Pregnancy in Rural England in Earlier Centuries," *Population Studies*, 20, 1966, pp. 233–243, and Philip E. Hair, "Bridal Pregnancy in Earlier Rural England Further Examined," *Population Studies*, 24, 1970, pp. 59–70; Gillis, *op.cit.*, pp. 20, 52, 19, 126–127.

16 *Ibid.*, pp. 140–141, 135–140, 110.

17 *Ibid.*, pp. 179–180, 219, 130.

18 *Ibid.*, p. 183. Britain did not reverse this anomaly until it passed the *Married Woman's Property Act* in 1882. In the Australian colonies, Married Woman's Property Acts were enacted by 1893.

19 *Ibid.*, p. 237.

20 *Ibid.*, p. 232.

21 *Pointers, Bulletin of the Christian Research Association*, March 1995, 5, 1, pp. 1–3.

22 *Ibid.*, pp. 18–20. See also Martin Ingram, *Church Courts, Sex and Marriage in England 1570–1640*, Cambridge Univeristy Press, Cambridge, 1987, *passim*.

23 Gillis, *op. cit.*, p. 135.

24 *Ibid.*, p. 196. Only Quakers and Jews were exempt from the provisions of the *Hardwicke Act*.

25 *Ibid.*

CHAPTER 2

1 For a valuable survey of the writings of Paul on women and an assessment of the impact of those writings, see Brendan Byrne SJ, *Paul and the Christian Woman*, St Pauls, Homebush, 1988.

2 Nadine Foley, "Celibacy in the Men's Church," *Women in a Men's Church: Concilium*, 134, 4, 1980, pp. 26–39.

3 See my study *Women in the Church: The Great Ordination Debate in Australia*, Penguin, Ringwood, 1989; also Richard Leonard SJ, *Beloved Daughters, 100 Years of Papal Teaching on Women*, David Lovell Publishing, Ringwood, 1995.

4 See Ian Maclean, *The Renaissance Notion of Woman: A Study in the Fortunes of Scholasticism and Medical Science in European Intellectual Life*, Cambridge University Press, Cambridge, 1980.

5 Tertullian, *De Cultu Feminarum*, i. I, quoted in D. S. Bailey, *The Man–Woman Relation in Christian Thought*, Longman, London, 1959, p. 4.

6 Elizabeth A. Clark, *Women in the Early Church* (vol. 13 in *Message of the Fathers of the Church*), Michael Glazier, Delaware, 1983, pp.17, 205; Margaret Aston, "Segregation in Church," in W. J. Sheils and Diana Wood (eds), *Women in the Church: Papers Read at the 1989 Summer Meeting and the 1990 Winter Meeting of the Ecclesiastical History Society*, Blackwell, Oxford, 1990; Keith Thomas, *Man and the Natural World: Changing Attitudes in England 1500–1800*, Allen Lane, London, 1983, p. 43. See also Peter Brown, *The Body and Society: Men, Women and Sexual Renunciation in Early Christianity*, Faber and Faber, London, 1989.

7 For a full discussion of the "churching" of women, see William Coster, "The Churching of Women, 1500–1700," in W. J. Sheils and Diana Wood, *op. cit.*, pp. 377–387.

8 For a full discussion, see Marina Warner, *Alone of All Her Sex: The Myth and the Cult of the Virgin Mary*, Weidenfeld and Nicholson, London, 1976.

9 *Ibid.*, p. 74.

10 Quoted *ibid*, p. 73.

11 Peter Brown, *op. cit.*, p. 224. Brown's work provides an extensive and thorough examination of this subject.

12 *Ibid.*, pp. 213–240.

13 *Ibid.*, pp. 241ff.

14 This section on Augustine draws primarily on his writings in R. J. Deferrari (ed.), *Treatises on Marriage and Other Subjects*, in *The Fathers*

of the Church: A New Translation, vol. 27, Washington, 1955. D. S. Bailey, *op. cit.*, provides an excellent summary of Augustine's theology of marriage. See also Eric Fuchs, *Sexual Desire and Love: Origins and History of the Christian Ethic of Sexuality and Marriage,* Marsha Daigle, trans., Cambridge and New York, 1983; Peter Brown, *Augustine of Hippo: A Biography*, Faber and Faber, London, 1967.

15 J. T. Noonan, *Contraception: A History of its Treatment by the Catholic Theologians and Canonists*, Harvard University Press, Cambridge, Mass., 1965, pp. 119–135, provides an excellent summary of Augustine's attitude to marriage.

16 Noonan, *op.cit.*, provides the definitive study of the Church's attitudes to contraception.

17 John E. Lynch, "Marriage and Celibacy of the Clergy: the Discipline of the Western Church: An Historico-Canonical Synopsis," *The Jurist*, 32, 1972, 1 & 2, pp. 14–38, 189–212, provides a valuable overview of the celibacy issue. Numerous other writings on the subject have arisen from the recent unrest in the Roman Catholic Church. See in particular Charles Frazee, "The Origins of Clerical Celibacy in the Western Church," *Church History*, 41, 2, 1972, pp. 149–167; Bernard Verkamp, "Cultic Purity and the Law of Celibacy," *Review for Religious*, 30, 1971, pp. 199–217.

18 Samuel Laeuchli, *Power and Sexuality: The Emergence of Canon Law at the Synod of Elvira*, Temple University Press, Philadelphia, 1972, describes this synod and its canons.

19 *Ibid.*, pp. 96–97.

20 Sozomen, *The Ecclesiastical History of Sozomen*, London, 1855, pp. 47–48; Socrates, *A History of the Church*, London, 1844, pp. 53–54. The tradition of allowing married men to be ordained but not allowing men once ordained to marry remains the tradition of the Eastern churches. It is also subscribed to, in very limited form, by the contemporary Roman Catholic Church, which has, in recent years, allowed the ordination of some married Anglican priests who have converted. A lobby group formed in England in 1977, the Movement for the Ordination of Married Men, proposed a full-scale reintroduction of this ancient permission, but did not support the marriage of men after ordination.

21 J. C. Ayer, *A Source Book for Ancient Church History from the Apostolic Age to the Close of the Conciliar Period*, New York, 1926, pp. 415–416.

22 Gerard Sloyan, "Biblical and Patristic Motives for Celibacy of Church Ministers," *Concilium*, 8, 8, 1972, p. 28.

23 The reference to the separation, and the commentary on it, are found in *The Babylonian Talmud*, I. Epstein (ed.), London, 1938, Seder Mo'ed, *Yoma*, pp. 1, 2, 11, 23, 24. Jacob Neusner has pointed out that, for the Jews, menstruation was a cause for far greater concern in matters of ritual purity than was sexual activity: *The Idea of Purity in Ancient Judaism: The Haskell Lectures, 1972–1973*, Leiden, 1973, p. 20. On the taboo against menstrual blood, see Clara Maria Henning, "Canon Law and the Battle of the Sexes," in *Religion and Sexism: Images of Woman in the Jewish and Christian Traditions*, Rosemary Radford Ruether (ed.), New York, 1974, pp. 272–3.

24 Brian Brennan, "Episcopae: Bishops' Wives Viewed in Sixth Century Gaul," *Church History*, 54, 3, 1985, p. 313–323.

25 Lynch, *op. cit.*, pp. 190–192. Damian's opponent, Ulric of Imola, maintained however that clerical marriage was the only way to control clerical immorality.

26 Lynch, *op. cit.*, pp. 197, 189–190: C. N. L. Brooke, "Gregorian Reform in Action: Clerical Marriage in England, 1050–1200," *The Cambridge Historical Journal*, 12, 1, 1956, pp. 4–5.

27 Edward L. Johnson and Andrew J. Weidekamp, "The Crisis of Celibacy at the Council of Trent," *Resonance*, 5, 3, 1966, pp. 45–72; Lynch, *op. cit.*, p. 209.

28 Bernard Verkamp, *op. cit.*, pp. 199–217.

29 Pope Pius XII quoted these words in his 1954 encyclical on priestly celibacy; Verkamp, *op. cit.*, p. 217.

30 Verkamp, *op. cit.*, p. 207.

31 Paul Collins, *Mixed Blessings: John Paul II and the Church of the Eighties – the Crisis in World Catholicism and the Australian Church*, Penguin, Ringwood, 1986, p. 77.

32 Thomas N. Tentler, *Sin and Confession on the Eve of the Reformation*, Princeton University Press, Princeton, New Jersey, 1977, pp. 186, 231–232.

33 Geoffrey Chaucer, *The Works of Geoffrey Chaucer*, F. N. Robinson (ed.), second edn, Oxford University Press, London, 1966, pp. 765ff.

34 Chaucer, *The Parson's Tale*, line 860.

35 *Ibid.*, lines 900ff.

36 *Ibid.*, lines 937, 930ff, 925ff.

37 Chaucer, *The Wife of Bath's Prologue*, lines 51–52, in *The Canterbury Tales*, Nevill Coghill (ed.), Allen Lane, London, 1977.

38 *Ibid.*, lines 149–162.

CHAPTER 3

1 J. T. Noonan, *Contraception: A History of its Treatment by the Catholic Theologians and Canonists*, rev. edn, Harvard University Press, Cambridge, Mass., 1986, pp. 306–311.

2 John Colet, *An Exposition of St Paul's First Epistle to the Corinthians*, trans. J. H. Lupton, G. Bell, London, 1874, p. 53. Details of Colet's life are recorded in D. Erasmus, *The Lives of Jehan Vitrier and John Colet*, trans. J. H. Lupton, G. Bell, London, 1883, pp. 31–35.

3 Colet, *op. cit.*, p. 91.

4 Quoted in J. H. Lupton, *A Life of Dean Colet*, G. Bell, London, 1887, p. 135. St Paul's Cathedral, London, retains to this day the unusual spelling of "virger" (from the Latin *virga*, rod) rather than the more common "verger."

5 Desiderius Erasmus, *A Right Fruitful Epistle ... in Laud and Praise of Matrimony*, trans. Richard Taverner, Short Title Catalogue 10492 (*A Short Title Catalogue of Books Printed in England, Scotland and Ireland, and of English Books Abroad 1475–1640*, A. W. Pollard and G. R. Redgrave (eds), London, 1946, rev. edn 1976). The Short Title Catalogue dates this first English publication in 1536, but recent scholarship prefers 1532; E.J. Devereux, *Renaissance English Translations of Erasmus: A Bibliography to 1700*, Toronto, 1983, p.8. See also *Encomium Matrimonii*, J. C. Margolin (ed.), in Erasmus, *Opera Omnia*, Ordinis Primi Tomus Quintus, Amsterdam and Oxford, 1975.

6 J. B. Payne, *Erasmus: His Theology of the Sacraments*, n.p., 1970, p. 109, claims they are his views. However, note the distaste for marriage and sexuality revealed in his praise of virginity in his *Sermon on the Marriage at Cana,* in *A Sermon Made: By the Famous Doctor Erasmus*, Short Title Catalogue 10508, London, 1533?

7 Erasmus, *A Right Fruitful Epistle*, pp. Bii–Biiii.

8 *Ibid.*, pp. Bvii–Bviii.

9 *Ibid.*, p.Cviii; Bruce Mansfield, *Phoenix of his Age: Interpretations of Erasmus c.1550–1750*, Toronto, 1979, p. 41.

10 Erasmus, *op. cit.*, p. Cviii.

11 *Ibid.*, pp. Cviii, Av, Avi.

12 *Ibid.*, p. Di.

13 *Ibid.*, pp. Dii–Diiii.

14 *Ibid.*, p. Avii.

15 *Ibid.*, pp. Ciii, Dvii.

16 *Ibid.*, p. Cii.

17 Henry VIII, *Assertio Septem Sacramentorum (Defence of the Seven Sacraments)*, L.O'Donovan (ed.), New York, 1908, pp. 383–384. For an account of the controversy over the authorship of the *Assertio*, see Edwin Doernberg, *Henry VIII and Luther: An Account of their Personal Relations*, London, 1961, pp. 22ff.

18 Martin Luther, *Commentary on 1 Corinthians VII*, in *Luther's Works*, Hilton C. Oswald (ed.), Concordia, St Louis, 1973.

19 *Ibid.*, pp. 11–12. Modern commentators would dispute that Paul actually argued this, claiming rather he was responding to this view, which had been posed by his correspondents in Corinth.

20 *Ibid.*, p. 26.

21 *Ibid.*, p. 13; Martin Luther, *A Sermon on the Estate of Marriage*, preached in 1519, in *Luther's Works*, J. Atkinson (ed.), Philadelphia, 1966, p. 9; Martin Luther, *The Estate of Marriage,* in *Luther's Works*, Walter I. Brandt (ed.), Fortress Press, Philadelphia, 1962, p. 49.

22 Luther, *Corinthinans*, pp. 27–29, 11.

23 *Ibid.*, p. 25.

24 *Ibid.*, pp. 21, 53, 18.

25 Martin Luther, *An Open Letter to the Christian Nobility of the German Nation Concerning the Reform of the Christian Estate*, in *Works of Martin Luther*, trans. C. M. Jacobs, Fortress Press, Philadelphia, 1943, pp. 120–122.

26 *Ibid.*, p. 122; Martin Luther, *Exhortation to all the Clergy Assembled at Augsburg, 1530*, in *Selected Writings of Martin Luther, 1529–1546*, T. G. Tappert (ed.), Fortress Press, Philadelphia, 1967, p. 74.

27 Luther, *Corinthians*, p. 20.

28 Steven E. Ozment, "Marriage and the Ministry in Protestant Churches," *Concilium*, 8, 8, 1972, pp. 52, 42.

29 Richard Marius, *Luther*, Quartet Books, London, 1975, p. 206.

30 Henry VIII, *Assertio*, p. 396.

31 Henry VIII, *A Copy of the Letters Wherein … King Henry VIII … Made Answer unto … Martyn Luther*, Short Title Catalogue 13087, London, 1528, p. Bviii.

32 *Ibid.*, pp. Bviii, C.

33 Marius, *op. cit.*, p. 205; Thomas More, *Responsio ad Lutherum*, J. M. Headley (ed.), S. Mandeville, trans., in *The Complete Works of St Thomas More*, vol. 5, Yale University Press, New Haven, 1969, pp. 687–688.

34 Thomas More, *A Dialogue Concerning Heresies*, Thomas Lawler, Germain Marc'Hadour, and Richard C. Marius (eds), in *The Complete Works*, vol. 6, p. 652.

35 Gordon Rupp, *Just Men: Historical Pieces*, Epworth, London, 1977, p. 46.

36 William H. Lazareth, *Luther and the Christian Home: An Application of the Social Ethics of the Reformation*, Muhlenberg, Philadelphia, 1960, p. 23.

CHAPTER 4

1 The lectures survive in printed form in Peter Martyr Vermigli, *Of Marriage and Sole Life; Specially of Ministers*, in *The Commonplaces of the Most Famous and Renowned Divine Doctor Peter Martyr*, A. Marten (ed.), Short Title Catalogue 24669, London, 1583. The claims about the treatment he and his wife encountered in Oxford are recorded in Anthony a'Wood, *Athenae Oxioniensis*, P. Bliss (ed.), London, 1813 (reprint, London and New York, 1967) col. 328. See also Philip McNair, "Peter Martyr in England," in *Peter Martyr Vermigli and Italian Reform*, J. C. McLelland (ed.), Wilfrid Laurier University Press, Ontario, 1980, p. 101.

2 G. W. O. Woodward, *The Dissolution of the Monasteries*, Blandford Press, London, 1966, p. 33.

3 See John Bale, *The Acts of English Votaries*, part one, Short Title Catalogue 1270, "Wesel" (Antwerp), 1546, pp. 4, 9.

4 Robert Barnes, "That by God's Word it is Lawful for Priests That Hath Not the Gift of Chastity, to Marry Wives," in *Supplication Unto the Most Gracious Prince Henry VIII*, Short Title Catalogue 24436, London, 1573, pp. 330–331.

5 *Ibid.*, p. 312. While the quotation here is taken from the 1573 edition edited by John Foxe, it is faithfully reproduced from the 1534 edition.

6 D. M. Loades, *The Oxford Martyrs*, B. T. Batsford, London, 1970, pp. 149, 154; John Foxe, *The Acts and Monuments*, vol. VI, George Townsend (ed.), London, 1846, pp. 677f.

7 See discussion of Cranmer's marriage below.

8 A. G. Dickens, *The English Reformation*, B. T. Batsford, London, 1964, pp. 246–7.

9 Jasper Ridley, *Henry VIII*, London, 1984, pp. 329–331; *House of Lords Journal*, 31 Henry VIII (vol. I 1509–1578), pp. 109–116.

10 D. S. Bailey, *Thomas Becon and the Reformation of the Church in England*, Edinburgh, 1952, pp. 16–17.

11 Philipp Melanchthon, *A Very Godly Defence ... Defending the Marriage of Priests*, trans. George Joye (pen-name "Lewis Beuchame"), Short

Title Catalogue 17798, Antwerp, 1541; George Joye (pen-name "James Sawtry"), *The Defence of the Marriage of Priests: Against Stephen Gardiner*, Short Title Catalogue 21804, Antwerp, 1541. Other works published at the time include two translations of a "domestic" book by Heinrich Bullinger, which contained a section on clerical marriage: *The Golden Book of Christen Matrimony*, trans. "Theodore Basille" (Thomas Becon), Short Title Catalogue 4045.5, London, 1542, and *The Christen State of Matrimony ...*, trans. Miles Coverdale, Short Title Catalogue 4045, Antwerp, 1541.

12 Melanchthon, *A Very Godly Defence,* pp. Aii, Aiii, B, Bv, Bvii, Dviii.

13 Joye, *op. cit.*, pp. Bviii, Aiiii.

14 C. C. Butterworth and A. G. Chester, *George Joye (1495?–1553): A Chapter in the History of the English Bible and the English Reformation*, University of Pensylvania, Philadelphia, 1962, pp. 223, 205; Joye ("Sawtry"), *The Defence of the Marriage of Priests*, p. Aiii. Other reformers to decry episcopal sexual hypocrisy at this time were the exiled English priest and naturalist, William Turner, writing in his *The Hunting and Finding Out of the Romish Fox*, Short Title Catalogue 24353, Bonn, 1543; and the German reformer Martin Bucer, writing in his *Gratulation ... unto the Church of England for the restitution of Christ's religion*, Short Title Catalogue 3963, London, 1549.

15 John Bale, *English Votaries*, Short Title Catalogue 1270, "Wesel" (Antwerp), 1546. A second part (Short Title Catalogue 1273.5), published in London, followed in 1551.

16 Joye, *op. cit.*, p. Cii.

17 Letter from Chapuys to Charles V, 17 April 1541, 32 Henry VIII, in J. Gairdner and R. H. Brodie (eds), *Letters and Papers, Foreign and Domestic, of the Reign of Henry VIII*, H.M.S.O., London, 1898, vol. XVI, no. 733. See also J. Ridley, *op. cit.*, p. 331.

18 Foxe, *op.cit.*, vol. VIII, p. 58; H. Robinson (ed.), *Original Letters Relative to the English Reformation*, Parker Society, Cambridge, two vols., 1846–7, pp. 466, 535; Ralph Morice, *Anecdotes and Character of Archbishop Cranmer*, in *Narratives of the Days of the Reformation*, J. G. Nichols (ed.), Camden Society, London, 1859; Foxe, *op. cit.*, pp. 44, 58; Matthew Parker, *De Antiquitate Britannicae Ecclesiae*

Canuariensis, Short Title Catalogue 19292, London, 1572, pp. 392–393.

19 Matthew Parker, *A Defence of Priests Marriages*, Short Title Catalogue 17519, London, 1567?, pp. 351–353; 2 & 3 Edward VI c. 21, *Statutes of the Realm*, vol. IV, part I, p. 67, quoted in H. Gee and W. Hardy, *Documents Illustrative of English Church History, Compiled from Original Sources*, Kraus Reprint, New York, 1966, p. 367.

20 John Bruce and T. T. Perowne (eds), *The Correspondence of Matthew Parker, D. D., Archbishop of Canterbury, Comprising Letters Written by and to Him From AD1535 to his Death AD1575*, Parker Society, Cambridge, 1853, p.x; George Pearson (ed.), *Remains of Myles Coverdale, Bishop of Exeter*, Parker Society, Cambridge, 1846, pp.xii–xiv; Henry Christmas (ed.), *The Select Works of John Bale, D.D., Bishop of Ossory*, Parker Society, Cambridge, 1849, pp. viii–ix; Dictionary of National Biography.

21 Peter Martyr (Vermigli), *The Commonplaces of the Most Famous and Renowned Divine Doctor Peter Martyr*, A. Marten (ed.), Short Title Catalogue 24669, London, 1583, p. Qqv; Martin Anderson, *Peter Martyr: A Reformer in Exile (1542–1562) – A Chronology of Biblical Writings in England and Europe*, Niewkoop, 1975, pp. 499, 102.

22 See the advice given by Dr Redman at the time of the 1547 Convocation, quoted by Parker, *op. cit.*, pp. 351–353. Thomas Becon reports a conversation on the subject he claimed to hear at the table of Archbishop Cranmer, when a group of learned divines maintained that there was no vow in England, but merely "custom"; Becon, *The Book of Matrimony*, pp. Dcvi–Dcvii, in *The Works of Thomas Becon*, three volumes, Short Title Catalogue 1710, London, 1560–1564.

23 W. H. Frere, *The Marian Reaction in its Relation to the English Clergy: A Study of the Episcopal Registers*, SPCK, London, 1896, p. 47; E. C. Messenger, *The Reformation, the Mass and the Priesthood: A Documented History with Special Reference to the Question of Anglican Orders*, vol.II, Burns, Oates and Washbourne, London, 1936, p. 61; Foxe, *op.cit.*, vol.VI, p. 561; Henry Machyn, *The Diary of Henry Machyn, Citizen and Merchant Taylor of London From AD1550 to AD1563*, J. G. Nichols (ed.), Camden Society first series 42, London, 1848, pp.73–74.

24 Matthew Parker, *A Defence*, pp. 63, 24, 174, 14, 269, 17.

25 Injunction no. 29, printed in H. Gee and W. J. Hardy, *Documents Illustrative of English Church History, Compiled From Original Sources*, London, 1921, pp. 431–432.

26 J. Bruce and T. T. Perowne, *op.cit.*, pp. 146, 151ff, 148f.

27 *Ibid.*, pp. 156, 158.

28 *Ibid.*, p. 157.

29 Letters of Theodore Beza to Bullinger, 3 September 1566; Perceval Wilburn (undated), in *The Zurich Letters ... 1558–1602*, H. Robinson (ed.), Cambridge University Press, Cambridge, 1845, pp. 128f, 358f; Humphrey and Sampson to Bullinger, July 1566, *The Zurich Letters*, pp. 157–164. J. Strype, *Annals of the Reformation*, Oxford, 1824, (reprinted three vols, New York, 1966) vol. I, p.81, claims that Parker and other clergy found it necessary to have their children formally legitimated in order to avoid the problems of bastardy.

30 John Veron, *A Strong Defence of the Marriage of Priests*, Short Title Catalogue 24687, London, 1562?; F. de Schickler, "Le Réfugié Jean Veron, Collaborateur des Réformateurs Anglais (1548–1562)," *Société de L'histoire du Protestantisme Français Bulletin*, 39, 1890, pp. 437–446; Machyn, *op.cit.*, pp. 271–273.

31 Veron, *op.cit.*, pp. 17–19, 21–23, 25–27.

32 Parker, *Defence*, preface (unpaginated).

33 For example, see R. Hooker, *Of the Laws of Ecclesiastical Polity*, book V, Short Title Catalogue 13712.5, 1597.

34 F. G. Emmison, *Elizabethan Life: Morals and the Church Courts*, Essex County Council, Chelmsford, 1973, pp. 214–215; Roger Manning, *Religion and Society in Elizabethan Sussex: A Study of the Enforcement of the Religious Settlement, 1558–1603*, Leicester University Press, Leicester, 1969, p. 173; Patrick Collinson, *The Religion of Protestants: the Church in English Society 1559–1625, the Ford Lectures 1979*, Oxford University Press, Oxford, 1982, p. 106; Nicolas Sander, *De Origine*, pp. 279–280.

35 Joel Berlatsky, "Marriage and Family in a Tudor Elite: Familial

Patterns of Elizabethan Bishops," *Journal of Family History*, 3, 1, 1978, pp. 6–22. See also Anne L. Barstow, "The First Generation of Anglican Clergy Wives: Heroines or Whores?", *Historical magazine of the Protestant Episcopal Church*, 52, 1983, pp. 3–16; Mary Prior, "Reviled and Crucified Marriages: The Position of Tudor Bishops' Wives," in Mary Prior (ed.), *Women in English Society 1500–1800*, Methuen, London, 1985.

36 Collinson, *op. cit.*, p. 115; Berlatsky, *op.cit.*, p. 11.

CHAPTER 5

1 Robert Barnes, "That by God's Word it is Lawful for Priests ... to Marry Wives," *Supplication*, in *The Whole Works of W. Tyndale, John Frith and Dr Barnes*, John Foxe (ed.), Short Title Catalogue 24436, London, 1573, p. 310.

2 Philipp Melanchthon, *A Very Godly Defence, Full of Learning, Defending the Marriage of Priests*, trans. "Lewis Bechaume" (George Joye), Short Title Catalogue 17798, Antwerp, 1541, pp. Avii, Aviii.

3 John Veron, *A Strong Defence of the Marriage of Priests ...*, Short Title Catalogue 24687, London, 1562(?), book, p. 17. (Veron's work consists of a substantial preface, paginated with Arabic numerals, followed by the work itself, also paginated in Arabic numerals without distinction from the preface. To distinguish, page numbers will be identified as "book" or "preface.")

4 Matthew Parker, *A Defence of Priests' Marriages*, Short Title Catalogue 17519, London, 1567, p. 249.

5 Barnes, *op. cit.*, p. 311; Veron, *op. cit.*, p. 17.

6 "James Sawtry" (George Joye), *Defence of the Marriage of Priests*, Short Title Catalogue 21804, Antwerp, 1541, p. Aiiii.

7 Melanchthon, *op. cit.*, p. Avii; Barnes, *op. cit.*, p. 317.

8 Thomas Becon, *Book of Matrimony* in *The Works of Thomas Becon*, three vols, Short Title Catalogue 1710, London, 1560–64, pp. ccccclxviii, ccccclxix, ccccclxxi.

9 Veron, *op. cit.*, p. 2; Heinrich Bullinger, *The Christen State of Matrimony*, trans. M. Coverdale, Short Title Catalogue 4045, Antwerp, 1541, pp. xxv–xxvi.

10 Peter Martyr (Vermigli), *Of Marriage and Sole Life*, trans. and ed. A. Marten, Short Title Catalogue 24669, London, 1583, p. 197.

11 Parker, *op. cit.*, p. 140; Martyr, *op. cit.*, p. 202.

12 See, for example, Barnes, *op. cit.*, pp. 313, 323.

13 Melanchthon, *op. cit.*, pp. Bviii, Cii.

14 Martyr, *Of Marriage*, p. 202.

15 *Ibid.*, p. 199.

16 Martin Bucer, *The gratulation of the Most Famous Clerk M. Martin Bucer*, Short Title Catalogue 3963, London, 1549, pp. Dvi, Ki, Eviii, Fii.

17 Thomas Becon, *Book of Matrimony*, p. ccccclxvi.

18 *Ibid.*, p. ccccclix.

19 Barnes, *op. cit.*, p. 334.

20 *Ibid.*, pp. 310, 330, 336.

21 See Thomas Martin, *A Traictise declaring and Plainly Proving, That the Pretensed Marriage of Priests ... is No Marriage*, Short Title Catalogue 17517, London, 1554, which provides the most substantial extant English response to the reformers.

22 Martyr, *op. cit.*, pp. 196, 197.

23 J. Bale, *English Votaries,* Part II, pp. cxviii, lxxvii.

24 W. Tyndale, *An Answer to Sir Thomas More's Dialogue*, H. Walter (ed.), Parker Society, Cambridge, 1850, p. 163.

25 Martyr, *op. cit.*, pp. 198, 193.

26 Melancthon, *op. cit.*, pp. Cv–Cvi.

27 D. S. Bailey, *op. cit.*, p. 111; John Colet, *Treatise on the Hierarchies*, quoted in J. H. Lupton, *The influence of Dean Colet upon the Reformation of the English Church*, London, 1893, p. 37.

28 Barnes, *op. cit.*, p. 317; Bale, *op. cit.*, p. 29.

29 Veron, *op. cit.*, p. 55.

30 Melanchthon, *op. cit.*, p. Diiii; Bale, *The Apology of John Bale Against*

a Rank Papist, Short Title Catalogue 1275, London, 1550?, p. lxxv.

31 Tyndale, *Obedience of a Christian Man*, 1528, in *Doctrinal Treatises and Introductions*, H. Walter (ed.), Parker Society, Cambridge, 1850, p. 230.

32 Tyndale, *An Answer to Sir Thomas More's Dialogue*, p. 158.

33 The 1550 Ordinal can be found in E. C. S. Gibson, *The First and Second Prayer Books of Edward VI*, J. M. Dent, London, 1910, pp. 308ff. F. E. Brightman, *The English Rite, Being a Synopsis of the Sources and Revisions of the Book of Common Prayer*, London, 1915, vol. 1, p. cxxxv. For a useful discussion of the origins of the Ordinal and Bucer's role in its development, see Paul F. Bradshaw, *The Anglican Ordinal: Its History and Development From the Reformation to the Present Day*, SPCK, London, 1971.

34 Barnes, *op. cit.*, p. 334; Bale, *Apology*, p. viii; Ponet, *An Apology*, p. xxviii; Ponet, *A Defence*, p. Aii.

35 Martin, *op. cit.*, pp. Aaiii, Bbii, Hliv.

36 Melanchthon, *op. cit.*, p. Bviii.

37 Book of Common Prayer, "The Form of Solemnization of Matrimony." Kenneth Stevenson, *Nuptial Blessing: A Study of Christian Marriage Rites*, SPCK, London, 1982, p. 137, identifies Luther as the source of this innovation without making any connection with clerical marriage. But in the light of the English experience, its inclusion may well have had a significant double meaning for Cranmer and his contemporaries, so many of whom had been forced to separate from their wives so recently.

38 Martin Ingram, *Church Courts, Sex and Marriage in England 1570–1640*, Cambridge University Press, Cambridge, 1987, p. 152.

39 *Ibid.*, pp. 153–157.

40 Martin Bucer, *De Regno Christi (De Royaume De Jesus-Christ)*, Francois Wendel (ed.), Paris, 1954 (vol. 15, *Martin Buceri Opera Latina*), p. 227; Martin Bucer, *Censura*, printed in E. C. Whitaker, *Martin Bucer and the Book of Common Prayer*, Essex, 1974, pp. 120–122.

41 See *A Prayer Book for Australia*, 1995, pp. 657ff.

CHAPTER 6

1 Edward L. Johnson and Andrew J. Weidekamp, *op. cit.*, pp. 45–72; *The Catechism of the Council of Trent*, trans. T. A. Buckley, London, 1852, pp. 332–350.

2 See Kathleen M. Davies, "Continuity and Change in Literary Advice on Marriage," in R. B. Outhwaite, *Marriage and Society: Studies in the Social History of Marriage*, Europa, London, 1981.

3 *The Oxford Book of Prayer*, George Appleton (ed.), Oxford University Press, Oxford, 1985, p. 82.

4 R. Barnes, *A Supplication Made by Robert Barnes Unto Henry the Eighth*, Short Title Catalogue 24436, London, 1573, p. 315; J. Bale, *The Acts of English Votaries ...*, Part II, Short Title Catalogue 1273.5, London, 1551, p. cxviii; W. Tyndale, *An Answer to Sir Thomas More's Dialogue*, H. Walter (ed.), Parker Society, Cambridge, 1850, p.153.

5 P. Martyr, *The Commonplaces*, trans. and ed. A. Marten, Short Title Catalogue 24669, London, 1583, p. 379.

6 J. Bale, *The Acts,* pp. 3, 24,30, part II, p. cxviii; *The Apology of John Bale*, p. xxxviii.

7 P. Melanchthon, *op. cit.*, p. Cviii-D.

8 "Sawtry," *The Defence of the Marriage of Priests*, pp. Cii–Ciii.

9 Martin Bucer, *Censura*, printed in E.C.Whitaker, *op. cit.*, pp. 120–122.

10 See "A Service for Marriage" (Second Form), *An Australian Prayer Book*, The Standing Committee of the General Synod of the Church of England in Australia, Sydney, 1978, and "A Service for Marriage" (First and Second Orders), *A Prayer Book for Australia*, E. J. Dwyer (Broughton Books), Sydney, 1995.

11 See James Turner Johnson, *A Society Ordained by God: English Puritan Marriage Doctrine in the First Half of the Seventeenth Century*, Abingdon Press, Nashville, 1970.

12 See L. William Countryman, *Dirt, Greed and Sex: Sexual Ethics in the New Testament and their Implications for Today*, SCM Press, London, 1989, pp. 149ff.

13 Roderick Phillips, *Untying the Knot: A Short History of Divorce,*

Cambridge University Press, Cambridge, 1991, p. 26. Much of this historical overview of the Church's attitude to divorce relies on Phillips' work.

14 Phillips, *op.cit.*, pp. 108ff.

15 *Ibid.*, pp. 65ff, 138.

16 *Ibid.*, p. 125.

17 *Ibid.*, p. 156.

18 *Ibid.*, p. 158.

19 W. J. Lawton, *The Better Time to Be: Utopian Attitudes to Society Among Sydney Anglicans, 1885–1914*, New South Wales University Press, Sydney, 1990, pp. 152ff.

20 *Ibid.*, p. 174ff.

21 See Muriel Porter, "The Christian Origins of Feminism," in *Freedom and Entrapment: Women Thinking Theology*, Maryanne Confoy, Dorothy A. Lee, and Joan Nowotny (eds), HarperCollins*Religious* (Dove), North Blackburn, 1995, pp. 212–215.

22 Phillips, *op. cit.*, p. 216.

23 T. A. Lacey and R. C. Mortimer, *Marriage in Church and State*, SPCK, London, rev. edn, 1947; A. R. Winnett, *Divorce and Remarriage in Anglicanism*, Macmillan, London, 1958, pp. 274–275.

24 *Putting Asunder: A Divorce Law For Contemporary Society*, SPCK, London, 1966, pp. 33ff.

25 *Marriage, Divorce and the Christian Church: The Report of the Commission on the Christian Doctrine of Marriage*, SPCK, London, 1971, pp. 71–73.

26 Under the terms of the Australian Church's constitution, canons are passed provisionally if they gain a minimum of two-thirds support in each of the three synod "houses" – bishops, clergy, laity. They must then be passed by each of the twenty-four diocesan synods in order to become law. If they fail to be passed in every diocese, they must return to another meeting of General Synod (generally three or four years later) for another two-thirds majority vote before they become law. Even then, they do not become law in any diocese until the canon is formally adopted by the diocesan synod.

27 See *Australian Family Briefings No. 3: Family Trends and Structure in Australia*, Australian Institute of Family Studies, July 1993. It is worth noting that, despite the high divorce rate, 53 per cent of married couples can expect to be together 30 years after marriage. That contrasts with the 41 per cent of couples who could expect a marriage of the same duration in the 1890s, when the divorce rate was below 1 per cent. Changes in life expectancy rates have created this little-noticed high level of marriage stability, and indicate that modern marriages are, on the whole, more stable than in earlier generations.

28 Phillips, *op. cit.*, pp. 255, 256.

29 For a comprehensive discussion of the Church's teaching on contraception, see John T. Noonan, *Contraception: A History of its Treatment by the Catholic Theologians and Canonists*, Harvard University Press, Cambridge, Mass., rev. edn, 1986.

30 Resolution 115, *The Lambeth Conference 1958*, SPCK, London, 1958.

31 *Ibid.*, p. 147.

32 *Marriage, Divorce and the Church*, SPCK, London, 1971, p. 72. Ramsey's article, "Christian Ethics in the 1960s and 1970s," is in *The Church Quarterly*, January 1970, pp. 221–227.

33 *Ibid.*

CHAPTER 7

1 Keith Rayner (Archbishop of Melbourne), *Human Sexuality: A Christian Perspective*, Anglican Media, Melbourne, 1994, p. 24.

2 *Something to Celebrate: Valuing Families in Church and Society*, The Report of a Working Party of the Board for Social Responsibility, Church House Publishing, London, 1995, pp. 116–118.

3 John R. Gaden, "A Christian Discussion on Sexuality," General Synod Paper No. 3, 1989, published in *A Theology of the Human Person*, Margaret Rodgers and Maxwell Thomas (eds), General Synod Paper No. 1, 1992, Collins Dove, Melbourne, 1992; Peter Corney, *Homosexuality: A Christian Response*, EFAC Victoria, no date.

4 See *The Briefing*, St Matthias Press, Sydney, 159–160, 20 June 1995.

The Briefing is a journal edited by the Revd Phillip Jensen, who represents the most reactionary Evangelical position within the conservative Diocese of Sydney. The edition quoted is a special double issue arguing against spiritual authority for women specifically on the grounds of these verses.

5 *Something to Celebrate: Valuing Families in Church and Society*, Church House Publishing, London, 1995, p.118.

6 *Issues in Human Sexuality: A Statement by the House of Bishops*, Church House Publishing, London, 1991, p. 41.

7 *Ibid.*, p. 36.

8 *Ibid.*, p. 44.

9 *Ibid.*

10 *Ibid.*, p. 28.

11 April Hyde, Margaret Rodgers and Michael Horsburgh, *A Godly Model: A Study of Clergy Marriage Breakdown in the Anglican Church of Australia*, draft, 1993, *passim*; *An Australian Prayer Book*, 1978, p. 612.

12 *A Prayer Book for Australia*, p. 786.

13 The debate is reported in the November 1993 edition of *SEE*, the monthly journal of the Anglican Diocese of Melbourne.

SELECT BIBLIOGRAPHY ▪

Specialist material not generally available, particularly the sixteenth-century tracts, have not been included in this select bibliography. Full references for such material can be found in the author's doctoral dissertation, "The Defence of the Marriage of Priests in the English Reformation," University of Melbourne, 1988.

BOOKS

Australian Institute of Family Studies, *Australian Family Briefings No. 3: Family Trends and Structure in Australia*, July 1993.

Bailey, D. S., *The Man—Woman Relation in Christian Thought*, Longman, London, 1959.

Bradshaw, Paul F., *The Anglican Ordinal, its History and Development from the Reformation to the Present Day*, SPCK, London, 1971.

Brown, Peter, *Augustine of Hippo: A Biography*, Faber and Faber, London, 1967.

Brown, Peter, *The Body and Society: Men, Women and Sexual Renunciation in Early Christianity*, Faber and Faber, London, 1989.

Bruce, John and Perowne, T. T. (eds), *The Correspondence of Matthew Parker, D. D., Archbishop of Canterbury, Comprising Letters Written By and To Him from AD1535 to his Death AD1575*, Parker Society, Cambridge, 1853.

Clark, Elizabeth A., *Women in the Early Church* (vol. 13 in *Message of the Fathers of the Church*), Michael Glazier, Delaware, 1983.

Corney, Peter, *Homosexuality: A Christian Response*, Evangelical Fellowship in the Anglican Communion, Victoria, n.d.

Countryman, L. William, *Dirt, Greed and Sex: Sexual Ethics in the New Testament and Their Implications for Today*, SCM Press, London, 1989.

Fuchs, Eric, *Sexual Desire and Love: Origins and History of the Christian Ethic of Sexuality and Marriage*, trans. Marsha Daigle, Seabury Press, Cambridge and New York, 1983.

General Synod of the Church of England, *Marriage, Divorce and the Christian Church*, The Report of the Commission on the Christian Doctrine of Marriage, SPCK, London, 1971.

General Synod of the Church of England, *Putting Asunder: A Divorce Law for Contemporary Society*, SPCK, London, 1966.

General Synod of the Church of England, *Something to Celebrate: Valuing Families in Church and Society*, The Report of a Working Party of the Board for Social Responsibility, Church House Publishing, London, 1995.

Gillis, John R., *For Better, for Worse: British Marriages, 1600 to the Present*, Oxford University Press, Oxford, 1985.

Hyde, April, Rodgers, Margaret and Horsburgh, Michael, *A Godly Model: A Study of Clergy Marriage Breakdown in the Anglican Church of Australia*, Draft General Synod Report, 1993.

Ingram, Martin, *Church Courts, Sex and Marriage in England, 1570–1640*, Cambridge University Press, Cambridge, 1987.

Issues in Human Sexuality: A Statement by the House of Bishops, Church House Publishing, London, 1991.

Johnson, James Turner, *A Society Ordained by God: English Puritan Marriage Doctrine in the First Half of the Seventeenth Century*, Abingdon Press, Nashville, 1970.

Lacey, T. A. and Mortimer, R. C., *Marriage in Church and State*, London, SPCK, rev. edn, 1947.

Laeuchli, Samuel, *Power and Sexuality: The Emergence of Canon Law at the Synod of Elvira*, Temple University Press, Philadelphia, 1972.

Lawton, W. J., *The Better Time To Be, Utopian Attitudes to Society Among Sydney Anglicans*, 1885–1914, New South Wales University Press, Sydney, 1990.

Leonard, Richard SJ, *Beloved Daughters: 100 Years of Papal Teaching on Women*, David Lovell Publishing, Ringwood, 1995.

Luther, Martin, *Commentary on 1 Corinthians VII*, in Hilton C. Oswald (ed.), *Luther's Works*, Concordia, St Louis, 1973.

Marius, Richard, *Luther*, Quartet Books, London, 1975.

Noonan, J. T., *Contraception: A History of its Treatment by the Catholic Theologians and Canonists*, Harvard University Press, Cambridge, Mass., 1965, rev. edn, 1986.

O'Day, Rosemary, *The English Clergy: The Emergence and Consolidation of a Profession*, 1558–1642, Leicester University Press, Leicester, 1979.

Phillips, Roderick, *Untying the Knot: A Short History of Divorce*, Cambridge University Press, Cambridge, 1991.

Porter, Muriel, *Women in the Church: The Great Ordination Debate in Australia*, Penguin, Ringwood, 1989.

Rayner, Keith, *Human Sexuality: A Christian Perspective*, Anglican Media, Melbourne, November 1994.

Stevenson, Kenneth, *Nuptial Blessing: A Study of Christian Marriage Rites*, SPCK, London, 1982.

Tentler, Thomas N., *Sin and Confession on the Eve of the Reformation*, Princeton University Press, Princeton, New Jersey, 1977.

Thomas, Keith, *Man and the Natural World: Changing Attitudes in England*, 1500–1800, Allen Lane, London, 1983.

Winnett, A. R., *Divorce and Remarriage in Anglicanism*, Macmillan, London, 1958.

ARTICLES

Aston, Margaret, "Segregation in Church," in W. J. Sheils and Diana Wood, (eds), *Women in the Church: Papers Read at the 1989 Summer Meeting and the 1990 Winter Meeting of the Ecclesiastical History Society*, Blackwell, Oxford, 1990.

Barstow, Anne L., "The First Generations of Anglican Clergy Wives: Heroines or Whores?", in *Historical Magazine of the Protestant Episcopal Church*, 52, 1983, pp. 3–16.

Berlatsky, Joel, "Marriage and Family in a Tudor Elite: Familial Patterns of Elizabethan Bishops," in *Journal of Family History*, 3, 1, 1978, pp. 6–22.

Blombery, Tricia and Hughes, Philip, *Australian Families: Practices and Attitudes*, Christian Research Association Research Paper No. 1, June 1994.

Brooke, C. N. L., "Gregorian Reform in Action: Clerical Marriage in England, 1050–1200," *The Cambridge Historical Journal*, 12, 1, 1956, pp. 1–21.

Carlson, Eric Josef, "Clerical Marriage and the English Reformation," *Journal of British Studies*, 31, January 1992, pp. 1–31.

"The Celebration of Marriage," *Pointers: Bulletin of the Christian Research Association*, March 1995, 5, 1, pp. 1–3.

Coster, William, "The Churching of Women, 1500–1700," in W. J. Sheils and Diana Wood, *op. cit.*, pp. 377–387.

Davies, Kathleen M., "Continuity and Change in Literary Advice on Marriage," in R. B. Outhwaite, *Marriage and Society: Studies in the Social History of Marriage*, Europa, London, 1981.

Foley, Nadine, "Celibacy in the Men's Church: Women in a Men's Church," *Concilium*, 134, 4, 1980, pp. 26–39.

Frazee, Charles, "The Origins of Clerical Celibacy in the Western Church," *Church History*, 41, 2, 1972, pp. 149–167.

Gaden, John R., "A Christian Discussion on Sexuality," General Synod Paper No. 3, 1989, in Margaret Rodgers and Maxwell Thomas (eds), *A Theology of the Human Person*, General Synod Paper No. 1, 1992, Collins Dove, Melbourne, 1992.

Henning, Clara Maria, "Canon Law and the Battle of the Sexes," in Rosemary Radford Ruether (ed.), *Religion and Sexism: Images of Woman in the Jewish and Christian Traditions*, New York, 1974, pp. 272–273.

Johnson, Edward L. and Weidekamp, Andrew J. "The Crisis of Celibacy at the Council of Trent," *Resonance*, 5, 3, 1966, pp. 45–72.

Lynch, John E., "Marriage and Celibacy of the Clergy – the Discipline of the Western Church: An Historico-Canonical Synopsis," *The Jurist*, 32, 1972, 1 and 2, pp. 14–38, 189–212.

Ozment, Steven E., "Marriage and the Ministry in Protestant Churches," *Concilium*, 8, 8, 1972, pp. 39–56.

Porter, Muriel, "The Christian Origins of Feminism," in Maryanne Confoy, Dorothy A. Lee and Joan Nowotny (eds), *Freedom and Entrapment: Women Thinking Theology*, HarperCollins*Religious* (Dove), North Blackburn, 1995.

Prior, Mary, "Reviled and Crucified Marriages: the Position of Tudor Bishops' Wives," in Mary Prior (ed.), *Women in English Society*, 1500–1800, Methuen, London, 1985.

Verkamp, Bernard, "Cultic Purity and the Law of Celibacy," *Review for Religious*, 30, 1971, pp. 199–217.

Yost, John K., "The Reformation Defense of Clerical Marriage in the Reigns of Henry VIII and Edward VI," *Church History*, 50, 1981, pp. 152–165.

MISCELLANEOUS

SEE (now *The Melbourne Anglican*), the monthly journal of the Melbourne Anglican Diocese, November 1993.

An Australian Prayer Book, The Standing Committee of the General Synod of the Church of England in Australia, Sydney, 1978.

The Book of Common Prayer, Collins, London (1662).

A Prayer Book for Australia, E. J. Dwyer (Broughton Books), Sydney, 1995.

INDEX

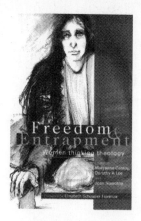

FREEDOM &
ENTRAPMENT

EDITED BY
MARYANNE CONFOY,
DOROTHY A. LEE &
JOAN NOWOTNY

"Feminist theology must ... articulate a spiritual feminist vision that affirms the dignity, self-determination, human rights, and well being of everywoman around the globe. *Freedom & Entrapment* both invites and challenges its readers to engage in such a critical feminist discourse, spiritual-religious vision, and struggle from below."

ELISABETH SCHÜSSLER FIORENZA

This important volume offers a collection of learned and insightful essays on Christian theology and feminism by leading Australian women scholars. The contributors explore the complex theme of "Freedom and Entrapment" from a variety of disciplinary stances, and in so doing enrich our understanding of the many threads of meaning that comprise the Christian outlook. This is not an exercise in the academic study of religion, but a vigorous engagement by the contributors from within their diverse Christian traditions: Anglican, Catholic, Protestant, Orthodox, and Aboriginal. Issues arising from church reform, gender and race relations, biblical exegesis, theological discourse, and feminist history will treat the reader to an invigorating experience of feminist writing at its best.

The contributors are: Veronica Brady, Patricia Brennan, Maryanne Confoy, Veronica Lawson, Dorothy Lee, Leonie Liveris, Joan Nowotny, Anne Pattel-Gray, Muriel Porter, Elaine Wainwright, and Erin White.

ISBN 1 86371 555 X

Dove
An imprint of HarperCollins*Publishers*

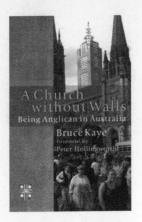

A CHURCH
WITHOUT WALLS

BRUCE KAYE

"This perceptive book does more than describe where Australian Anglicans have come from, though its historical perspective is immensely important. Dr Kaye calls us to engage with contemporary society in an invigorating reinterpretation of the Anglican commitment to incarnational theology. This scholarly and thoughtful study offers hope for a significant Anglican future in this country."

MURIEL PORTER

In *A Church without Walls* Bruce Kaye urges the Anglican Church to fulfil its historical mission in Australian society, to honor commitments to the nation that lie at the heart of an authentic Anglican identity. Bruce Kaye has written a book that will instruct and inform, as well as challenge and inspire. The rich heritage of Anglicanism, Kaye shows, can be restated in a modern vocabulary and rejuvenated to serve the needs of Australia today. These concerns form the basis of a fascinating discussion.

A Church without Walls should be read by all who care about the ecumenical possibilities of Christianity and about the religious orientations that have shaped, and will continue to shape, Australian society. This book is bound to provoke thoughtful discussion among people who are interested in the spiritual destiny and nationhood of Australia.

ISBN 1 86371 557 6

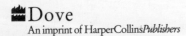

Dove
An imprint of HarperCollins*Publishers*